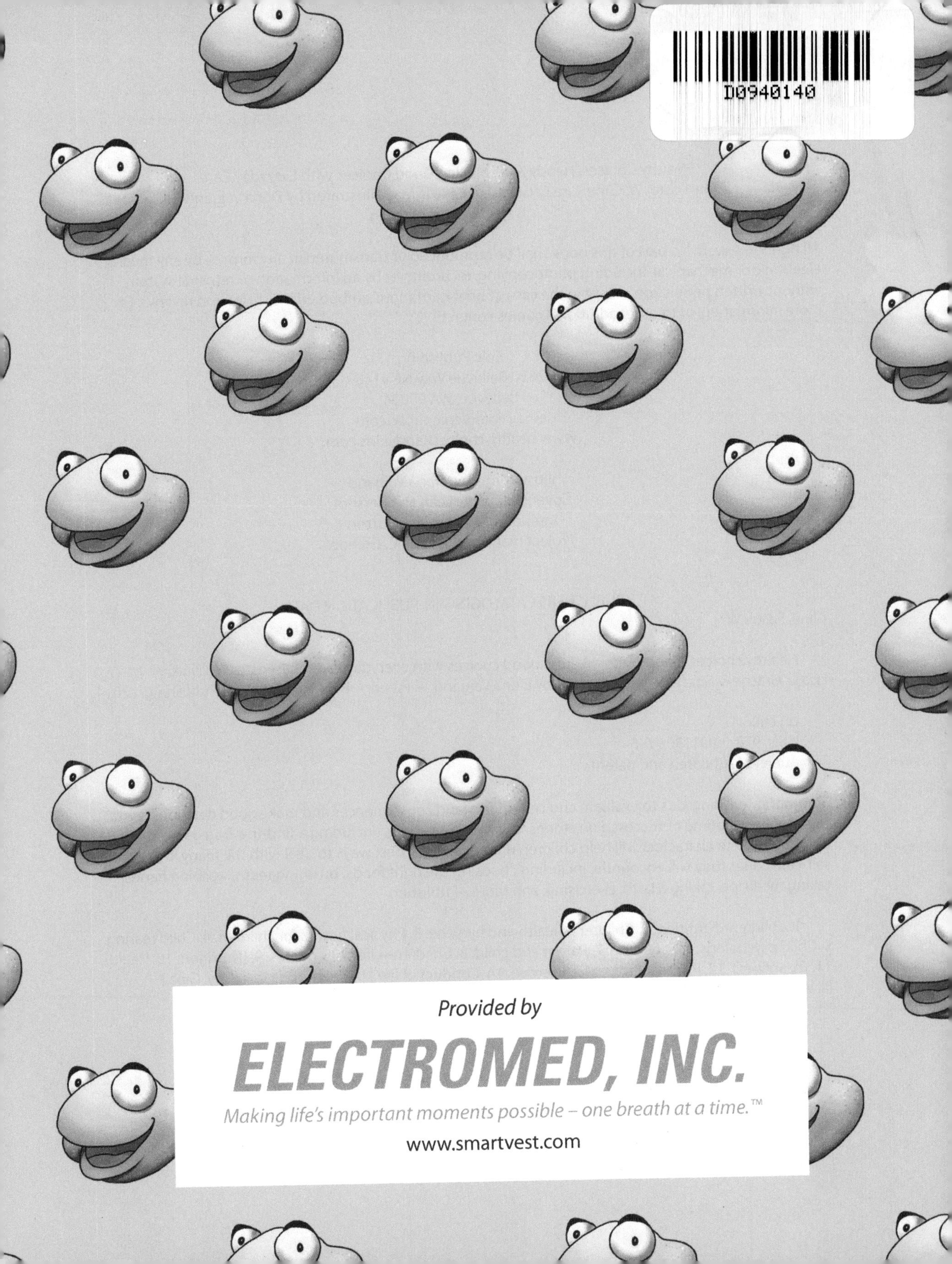
D0940140
Provided by
ELECTROMED, INC.
Making life's important moments possible – one breath at a time.™
www.smartvest.com

Healthy Choices, Happy Kids: Making Good Choices with Everyday Care
by Foster W. Cline, Lisa C. Greene & Gina L. May; illustrated by Dona Vajgand

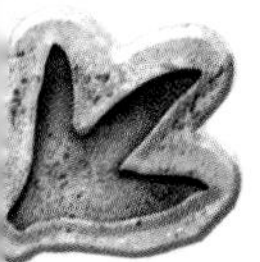

Epic Publishing
2620 Bellevue Way NE #146
Bellevue, WA 98004
email: info@epicpubllc.com
www.healthychoiceshappykids.com

Illustrations by: Dona Vajgand
Cover design by: Leah Hendershot
Interior design by: Lisa Norton
Project managed by: Lisa C. Greene

PUBLISHERS CATALOGING-IN-PUBLICATION DATA

Cline, Foster W.

Healthy choices, Happy kids : Making good choices with everyday care / by: Foster W. Cline, Lisa C. Greene & Gina L. May ; illustrated by Dona Vajgand. -- 1st ed. -- Bellevue, WA : Epic Publishing, c2014.

p. ; cm.
ISBN: 978-0-9911303-0-6
Audience: Children and parents

Summary: Teaching kids to evaluate choices, understand consequences and make good decisions is vital to ensuring a lifetime of success. Fun stories, colorful illustrations (including a find-the-frog game), and easy-to-relate-to characters will help children understand the best ways to deal with the many important self-care issues they will encounter, including choosing the right foods, brushing teeth, washing hands, taking medicine, taking a bath, exercising, and more.--Publisher.

1. Children--Nutrition. 2. Children--Health and hygiene. 3. Physical fitness for children. 4. Child rearing. 5. Child psychology. 6. Parenting. 7. Parent and child. 8. Children--Life skills guides. 9. [Nutrition. 10. Health. 11. Cleanliness. 12. Physical fitness. 13. Exercise. 14. Conduct of life.] I. Greene, Lisa C. II. May, Gina L. III. Vajgand, Dona. IV. Title.
HQ772.5 .C55 2014 2014931198
649/.1--dc23
1405

Published in the United States of America, May 2014
First Edition

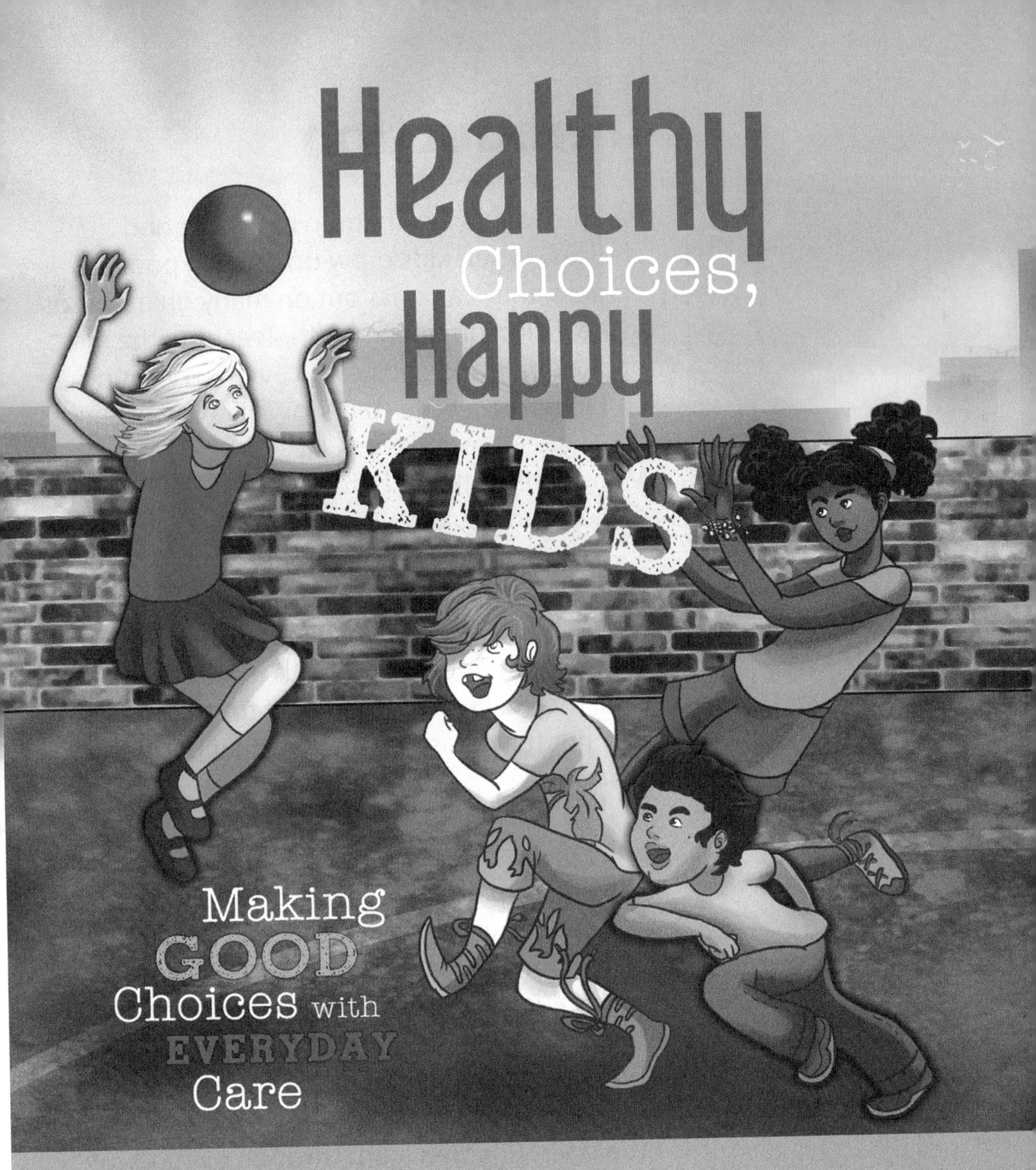

Foster W. Cline, M.D., Lisa C. Greene & Gina L. May
Illustrated by Dona Vajgand

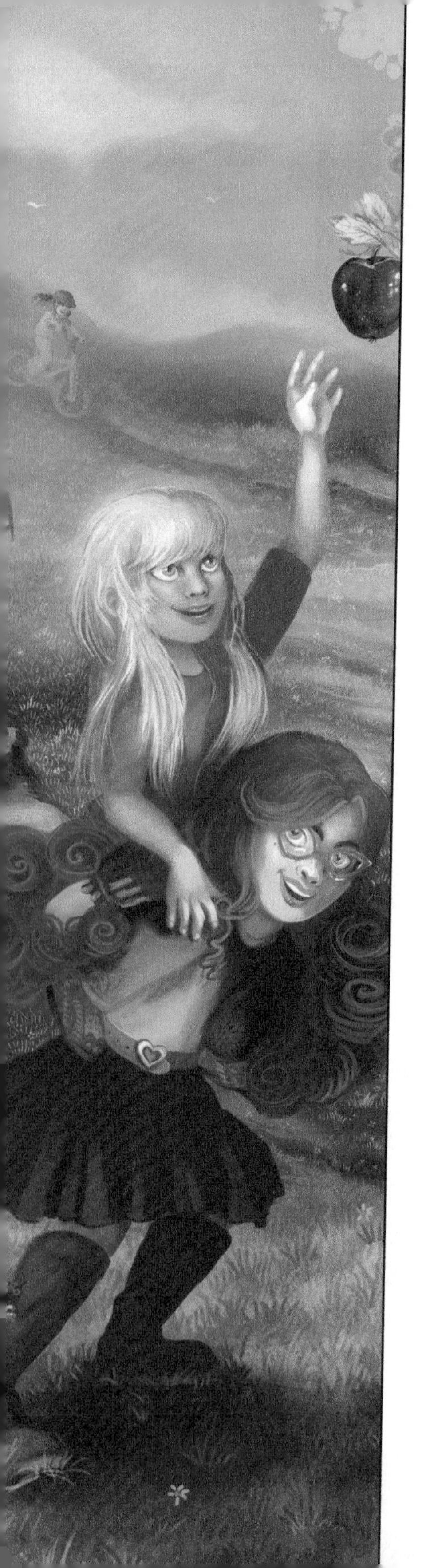

Introduction

Parents want their children to make good choices. When kids grow up making poor choices, they can miss out on many great things in life including good health. Teaching the idea of "making good choices" to even very young children can set the stage for a lifetime of success.

Many parents find it hard to teach little ones to make good choices. Why is this?

First, the results of poor choices may not appear until years later. Kids find it hard to connect not brushing their teeth now with tooth decay later. Until they have had the pain of tooth decay, they may not fully grasp the impact that poor choice can have.

Second, it can be hard to teach good, old concepts in a fresh, new way. You have a greater chance for success with kids when your teaching is fresh, fun, and even silly. Have fun with this book. Laugh, be funny, and ask questions.

Third, most parents *talk* about these issues with their kids, but talking does not work well with little ones. Children learn through pictures, by doing, and by watching the way you and other adults live your lives.

This book will help you teach your children about both good and bad choices. There are twelve scenes that represent common childhood issues. Each scene has three pictures: a neutral scene, a bad choice and a good choice. Have fun talking about what is happening in each scene. When your kids pop up on your lap, snuggle in, and talk with you about making good choices, they will connect wise choices with love and fun. You will "lock in" learning. The pictures help even young kids grasp the concepts.

Of course, actions speak louder than words. When you make healthy choices in your own life and talk about them with your child, you will have a winning pair!

We have added a bonus section at the end of this book to help you learn more about teaching your children to make wise choices about their bodies. Read it before sharing the book with your child.

We are certain that as you and your children have fun with this book, you will set the stage for success. Teach and model good choices early and your kids will be ready to be all they can be.

PS: Be sure to look for the frog hidden on each page.

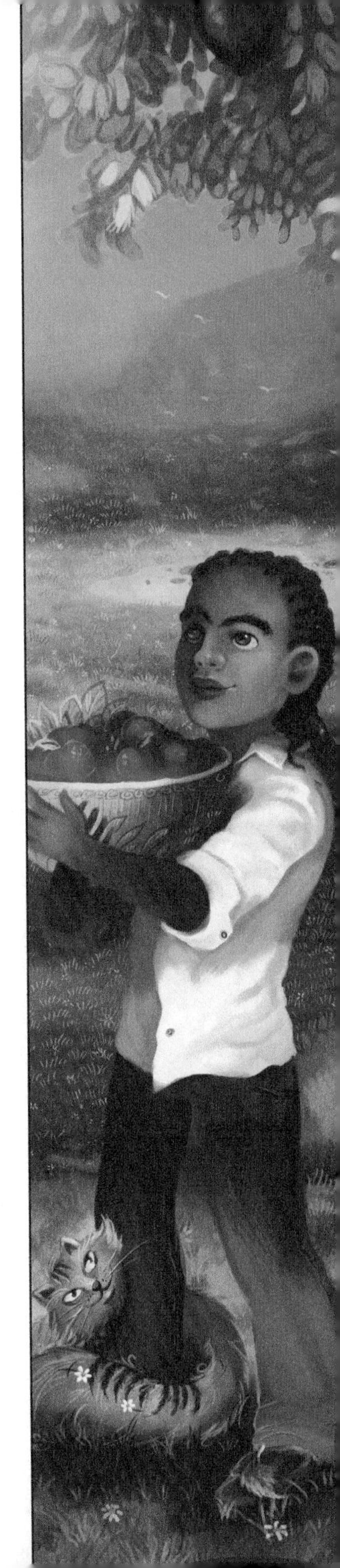

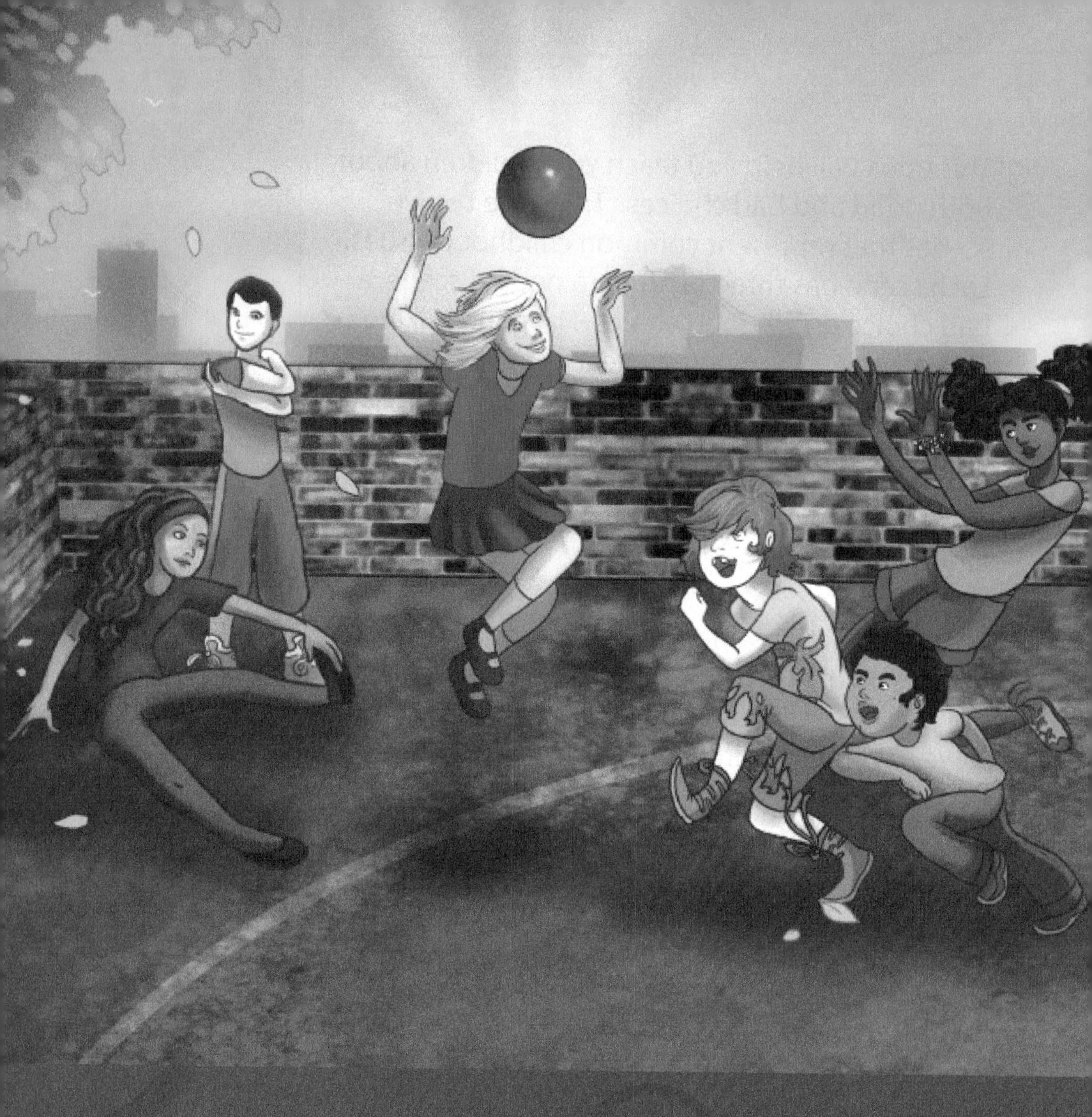

Meet the kids in our stories:
Rosa, Sam, Maddie, Elliott,

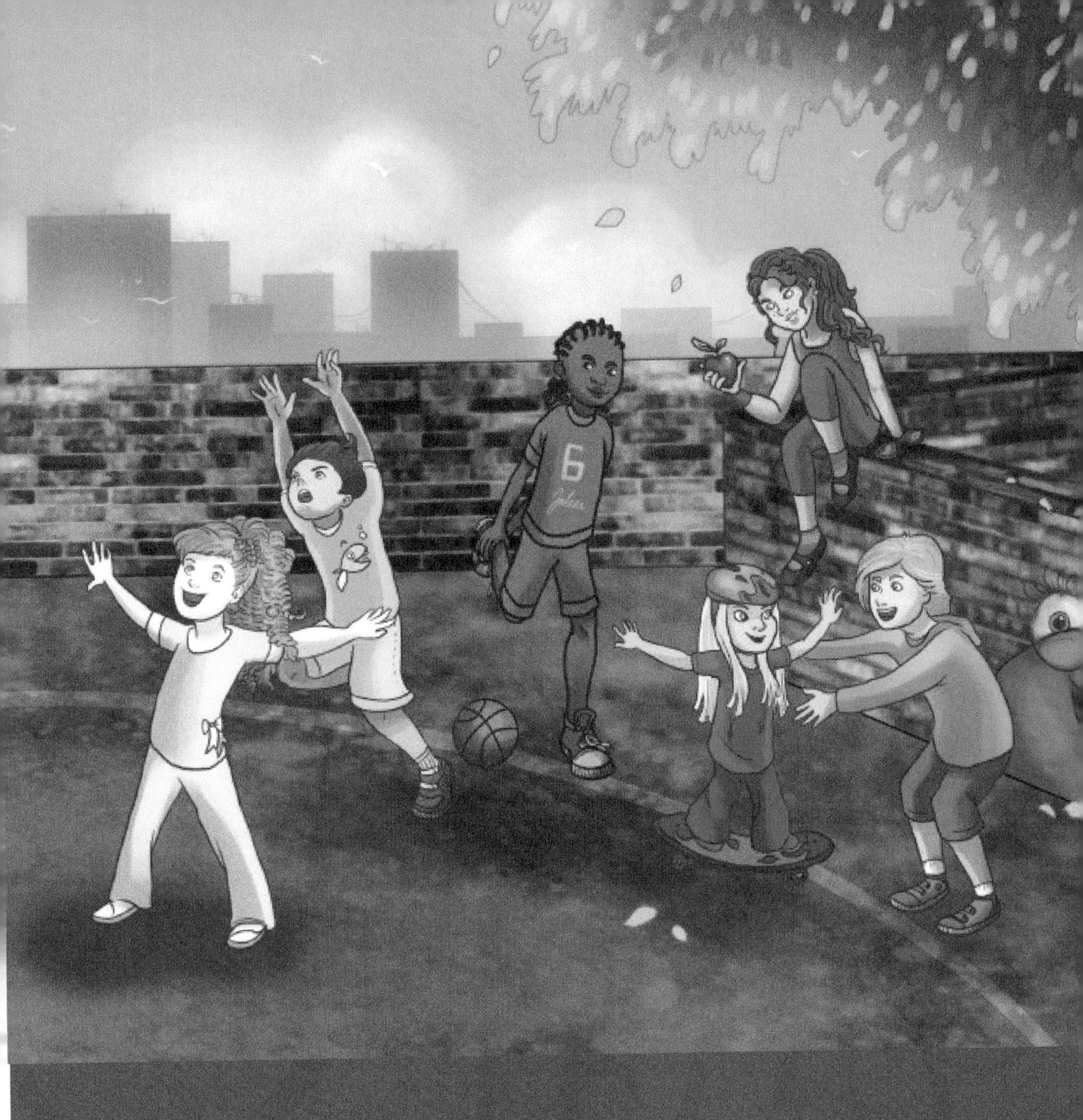

Aydin, Kayla, Katie, Nick,
Jalen, Kasey, Emily, and Jake.

It is time to eat.

Mom says,
"Nick, I made a
good meal for you."

Nick thinks,
"I don't want chicken."

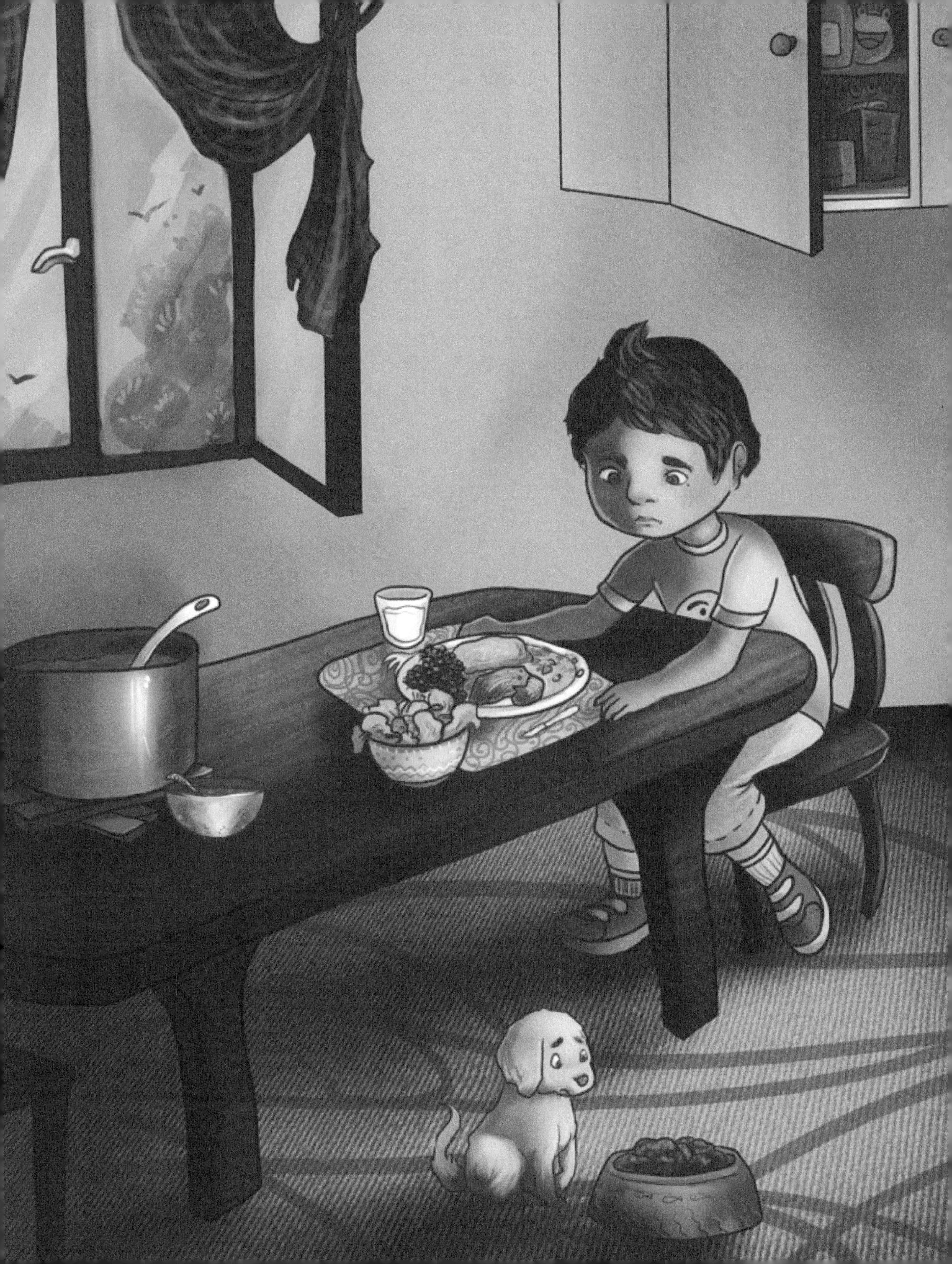

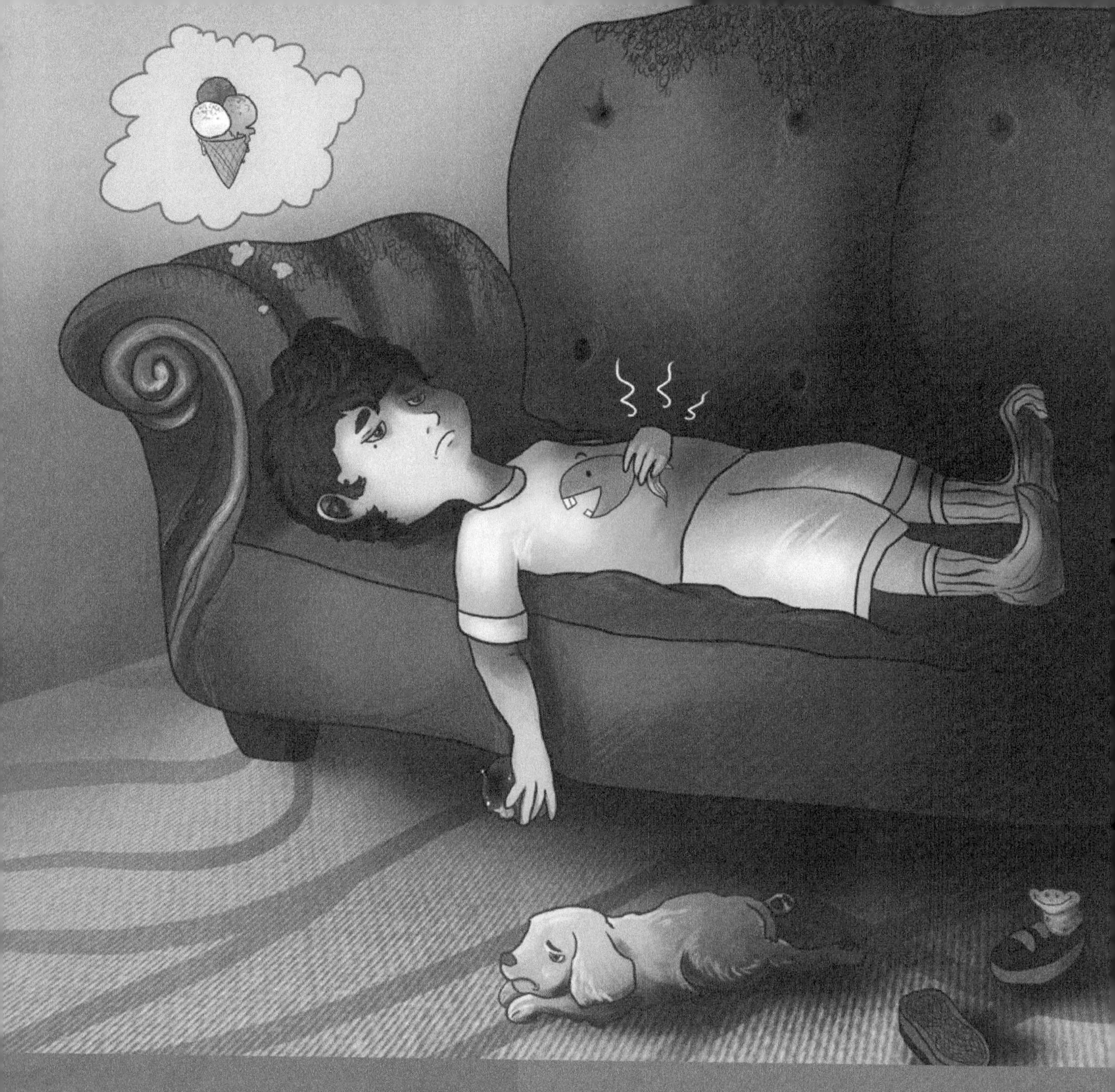

Nick does not eat his dinner.
Now he is very hungry.
Mom says, “Nick, you may have an apple.”
Nick does not want an apple.

Why does Nick wish he had eaten his dinner?

Nick tries some new foods. He finds that he likes them!
Mom says, “Nick, you ate a good, healthy dinner.”
Nick feels proud of himself.
His body feels good, too.

Nick likes to try new foods from the garden.
What new foods would you like to try?

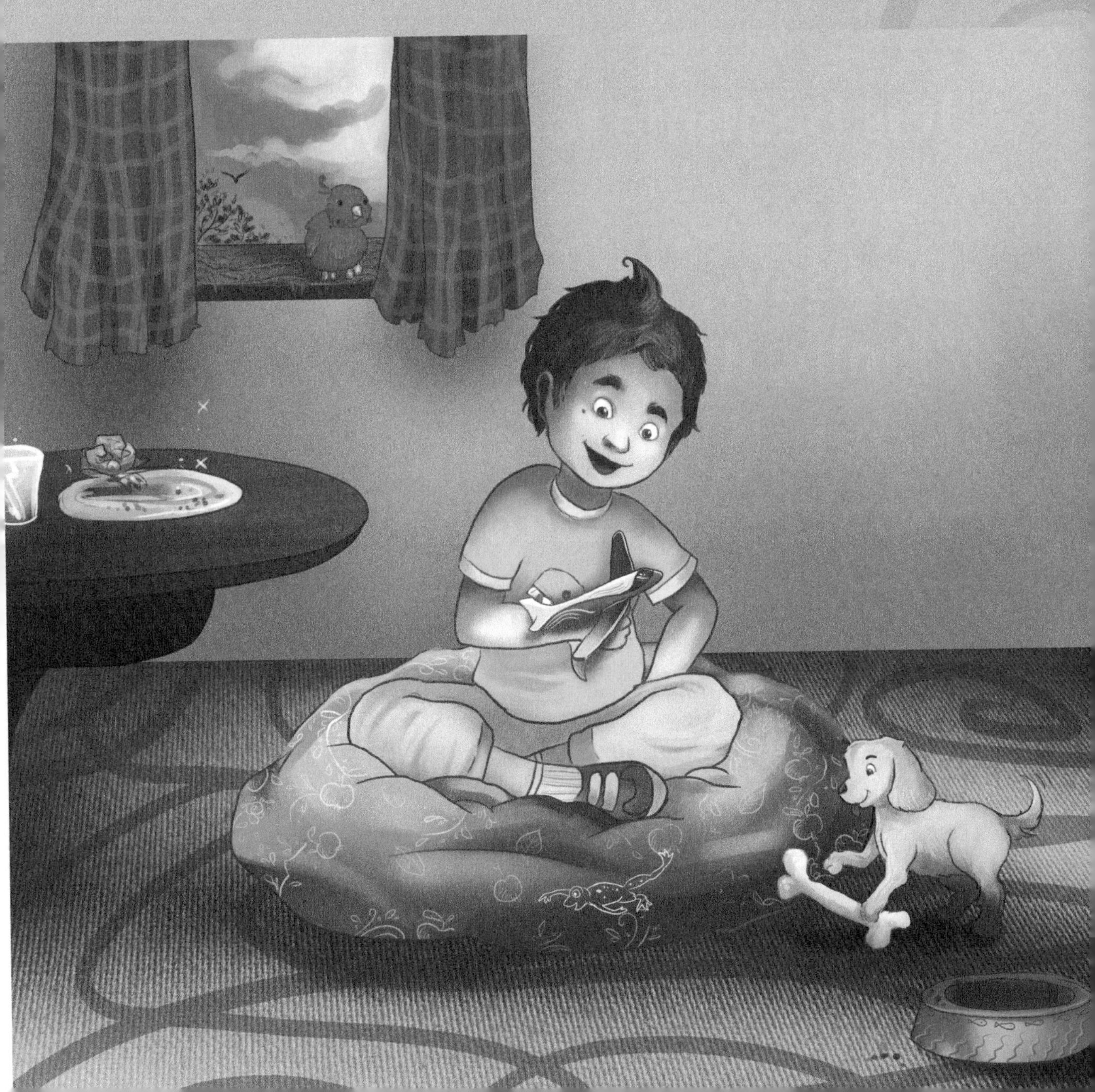

It is bedtime for Emily.

Dad says,
"Emily, it is time
to brush your teeth.
Would you like to brush them
upstairs or downstairs?"

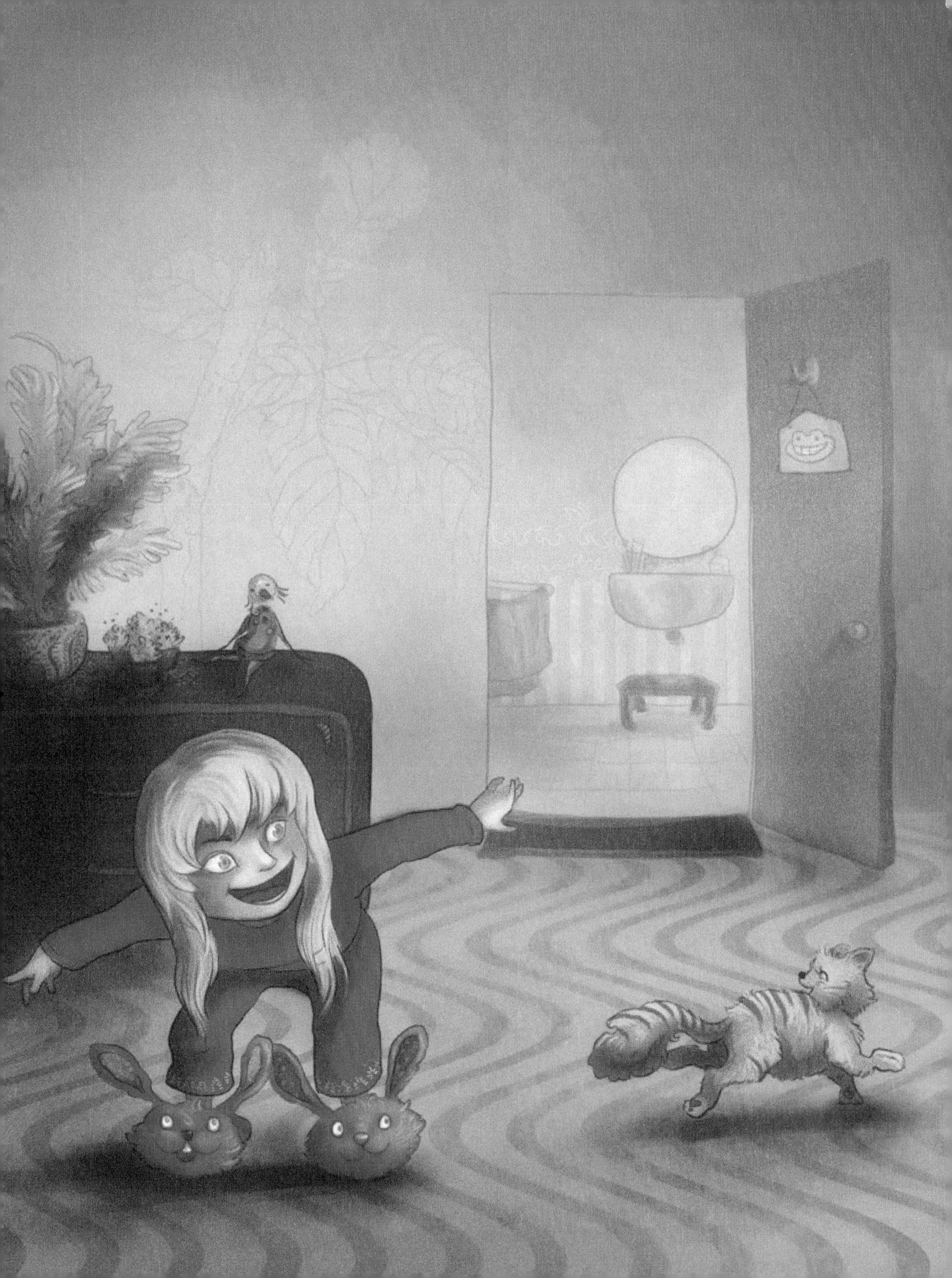

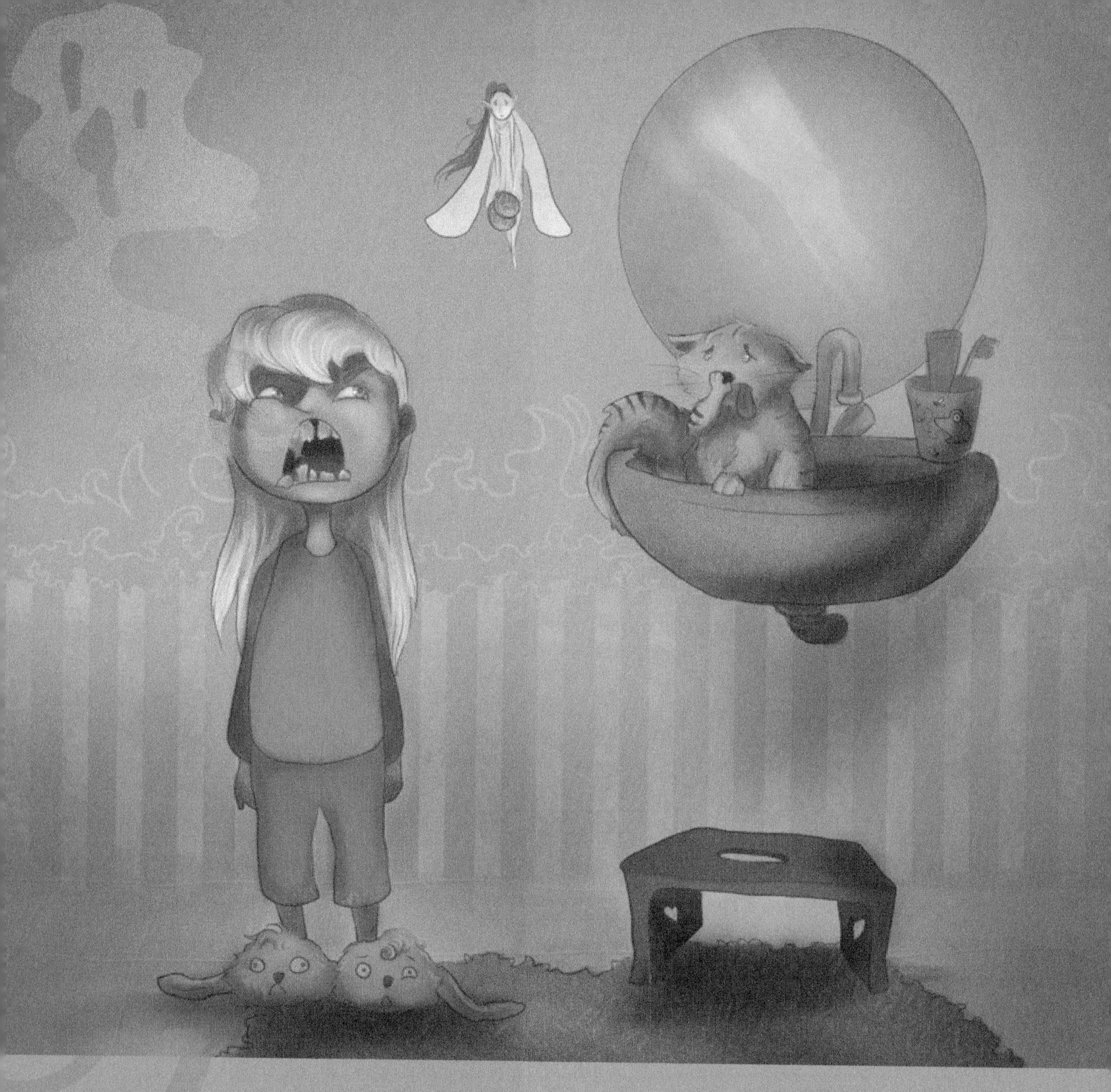

Emily thinks, "I do not want to brush my teeth."
Emily goes to bed without brushing her teeth.
Her teeth turn yellow and her breath smells bad.
Emily's teeth are so dirty that the tooth fairy
only leaves a penny under her pillow!

What has happened to Emily's teeth?

Emily says, "Okay, Dad. I will brush my teeth upstairs."
Emily brushes her teeth with her pink toothbrush.
Dad says, "Good job Emily. Your teeth look pretty and clean. Your breath smells good, too."

Emily likes to use minty toothpaste with her pink toothbrush. How about you?

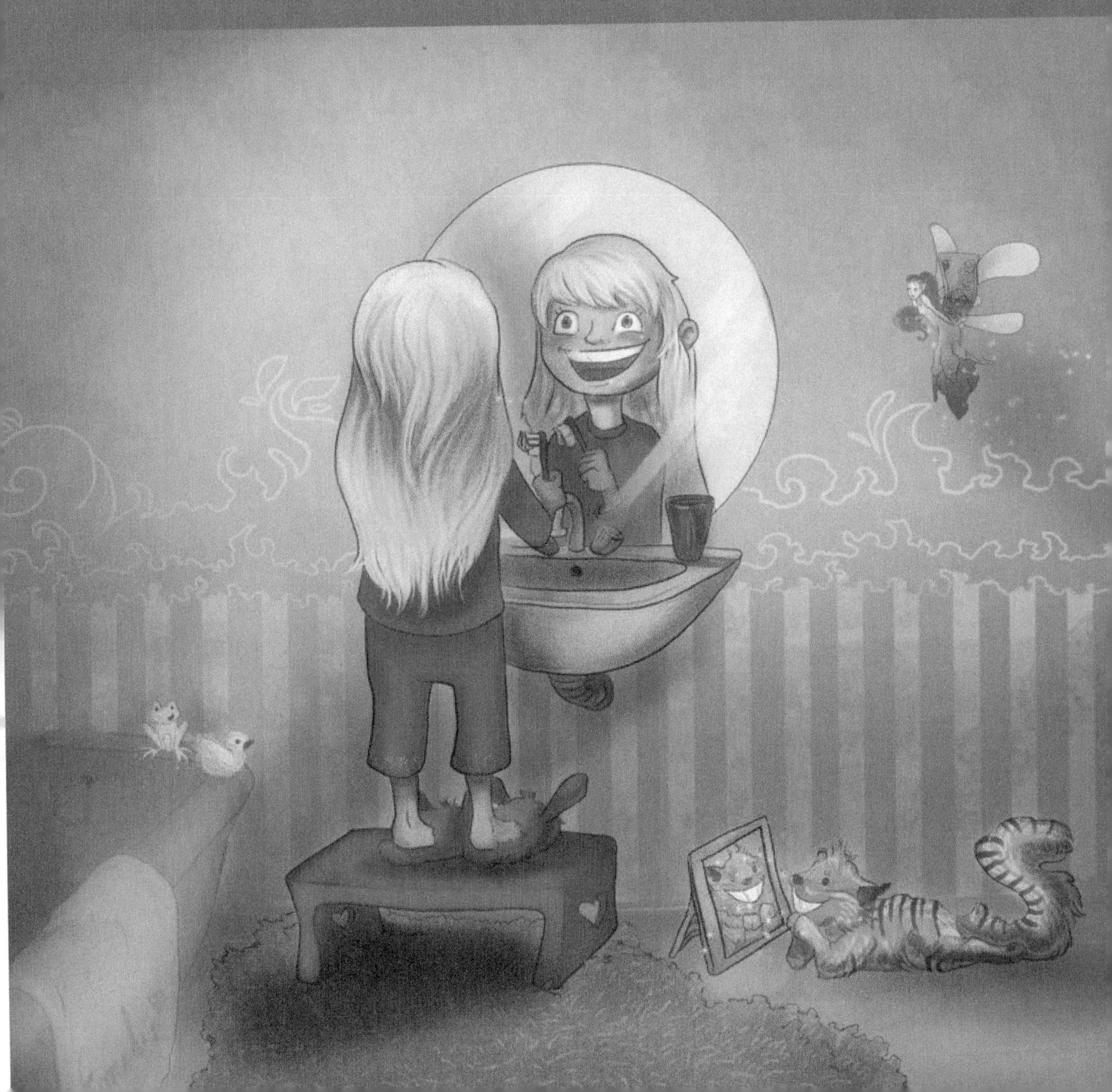

Sam has been playing outside.

When he gets home,
Grandma says,
“I am so glad you had fun!
Would you like a shower
or a bath before bed?”

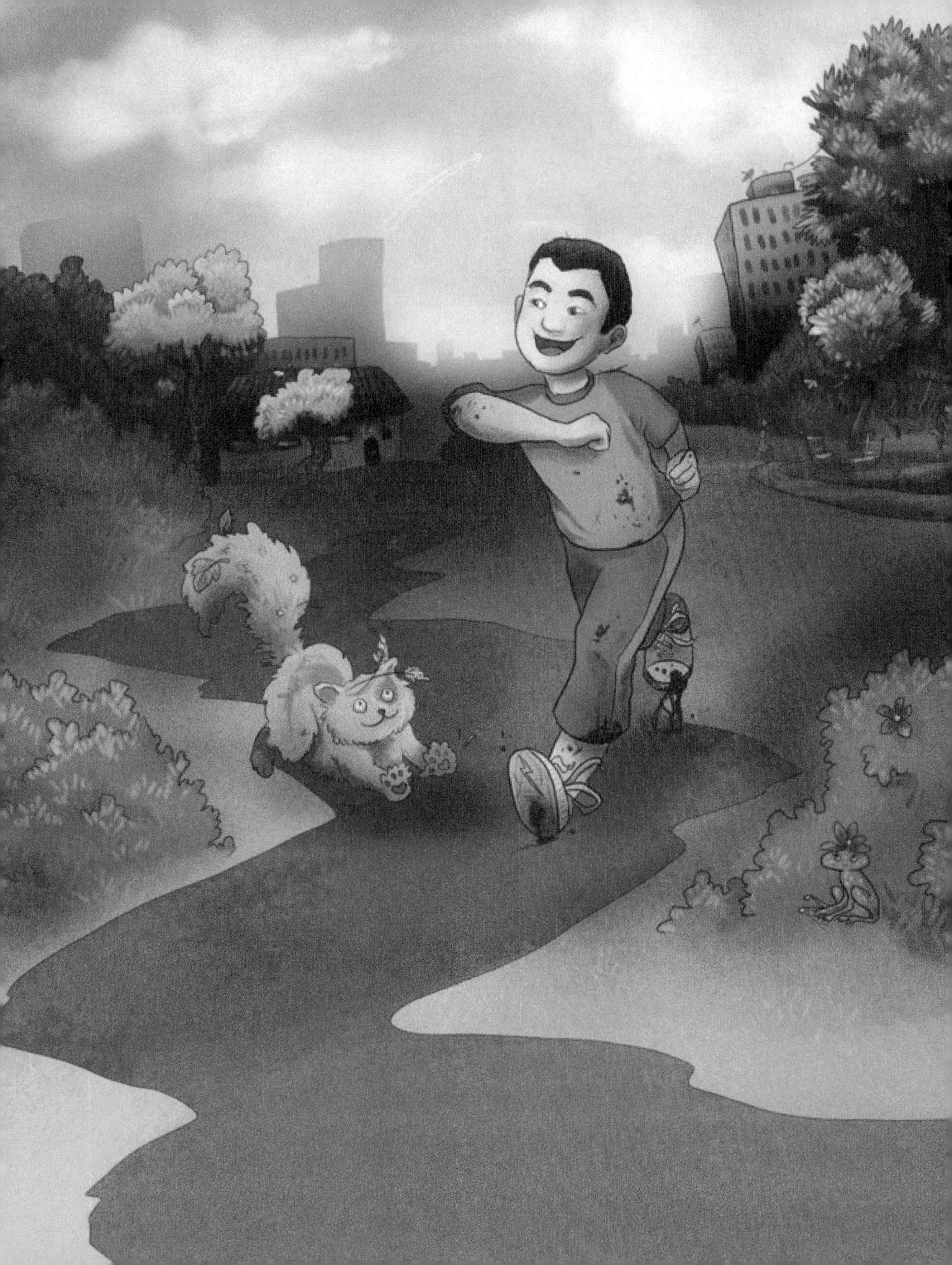

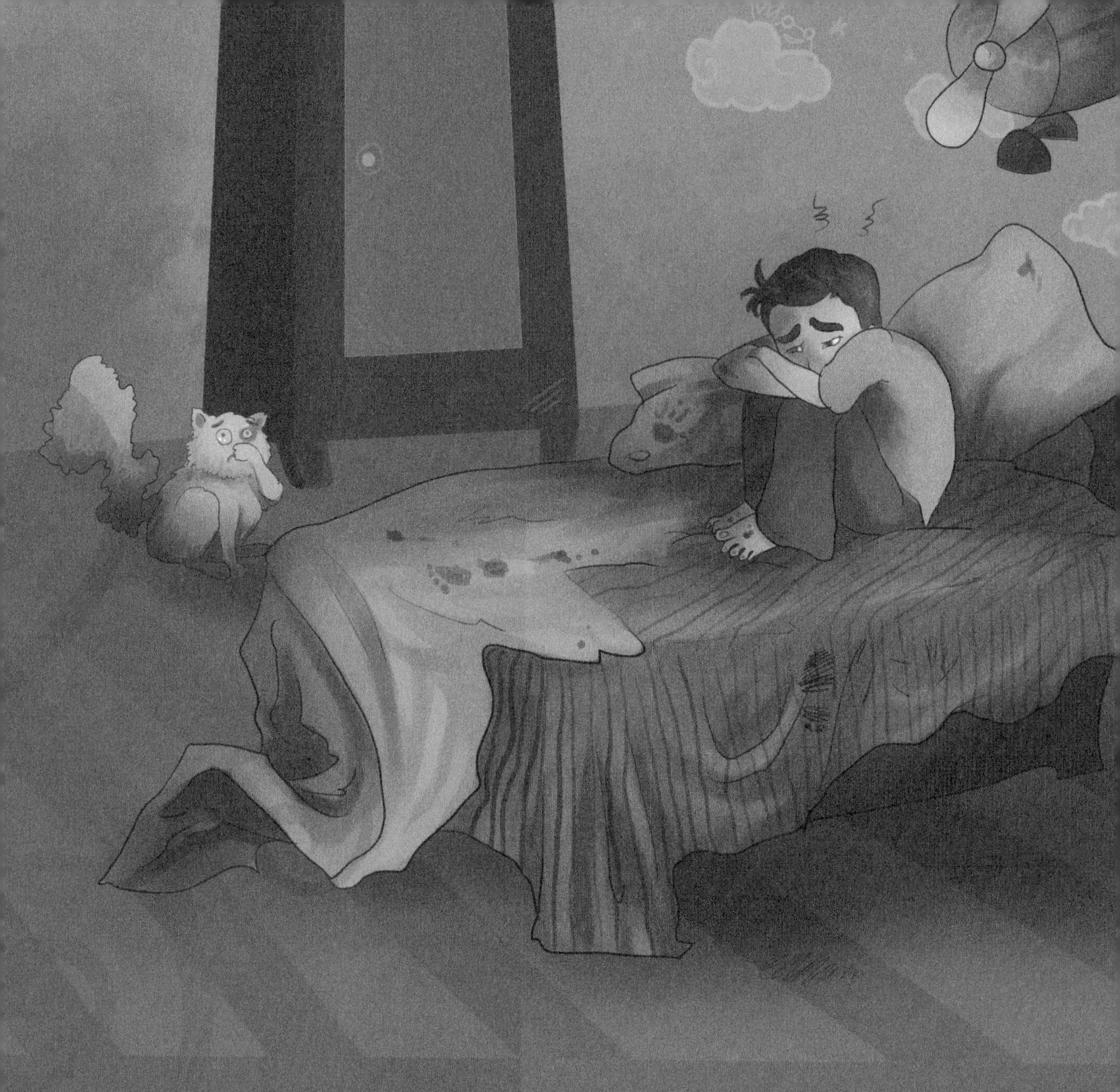

Sam does not want to take a bath or shower.
He goes to bed without one. Sam feels sticky and dirty.
The clean sheets on his bed are dirty now, too.
Sam will need to change them. Sam is so stinky
that even his cat does not want to sleep with him!

Why is Sam feeling sad?

Sam takes a nice warm bath. He washes his hair with his favorite shampoo. It smells like watermelon. Sam feels happy and clean. He crawls into bed with his favorite book. Sam's kitty cuddles up beside him. Kitty sniffs Sam and purrs. Sam must smell very good.

What is your favorite shampoo?

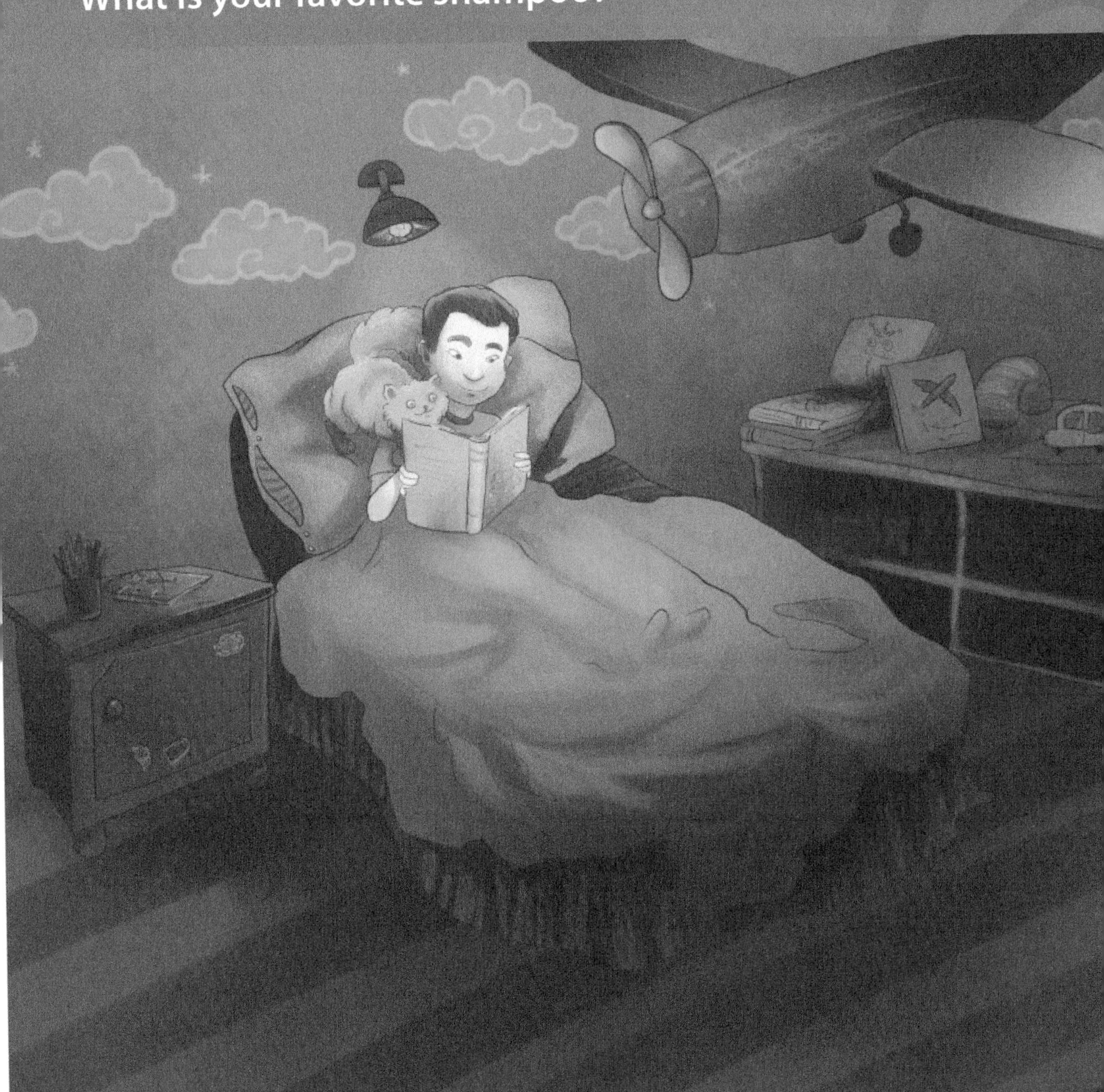

Katie is sick.

Mom says,
“Katie, it is time
for your medicine.
What would you like
to drink with it?”

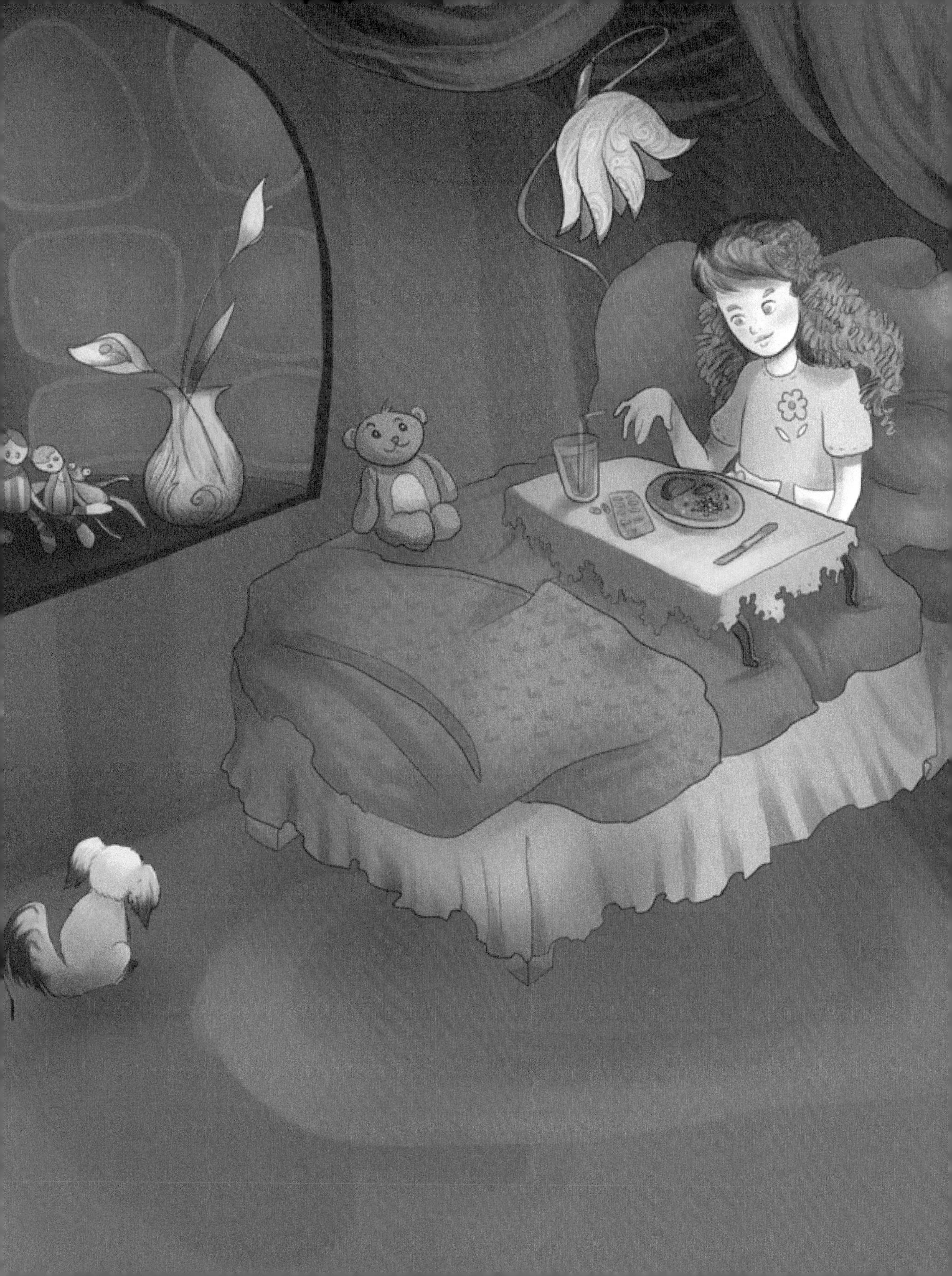

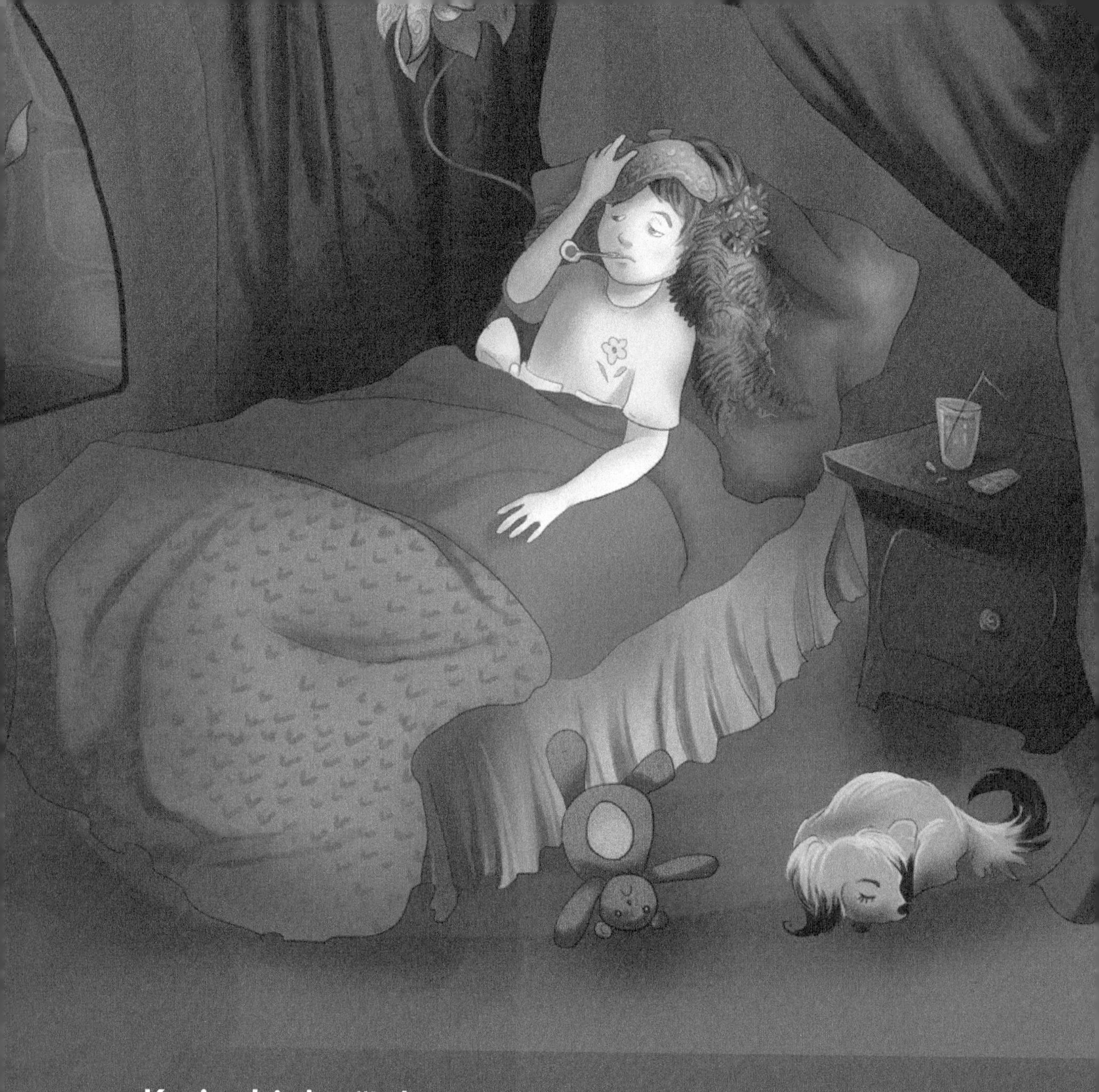

Katie thinks, “I do not want to take my medicine.”
She does not take it.
Her fever gets worse and her head hurts more.
She may have to go to the doctor to get better.

Why is Katie getting sicker?

Katie takes her medicine.
The medicine helps Katie's headache and fever go away.
She wants to get out of bed now.
She is ready to go play!

Katie likes to take medicine with apple juice
or ginger ale. What about you?

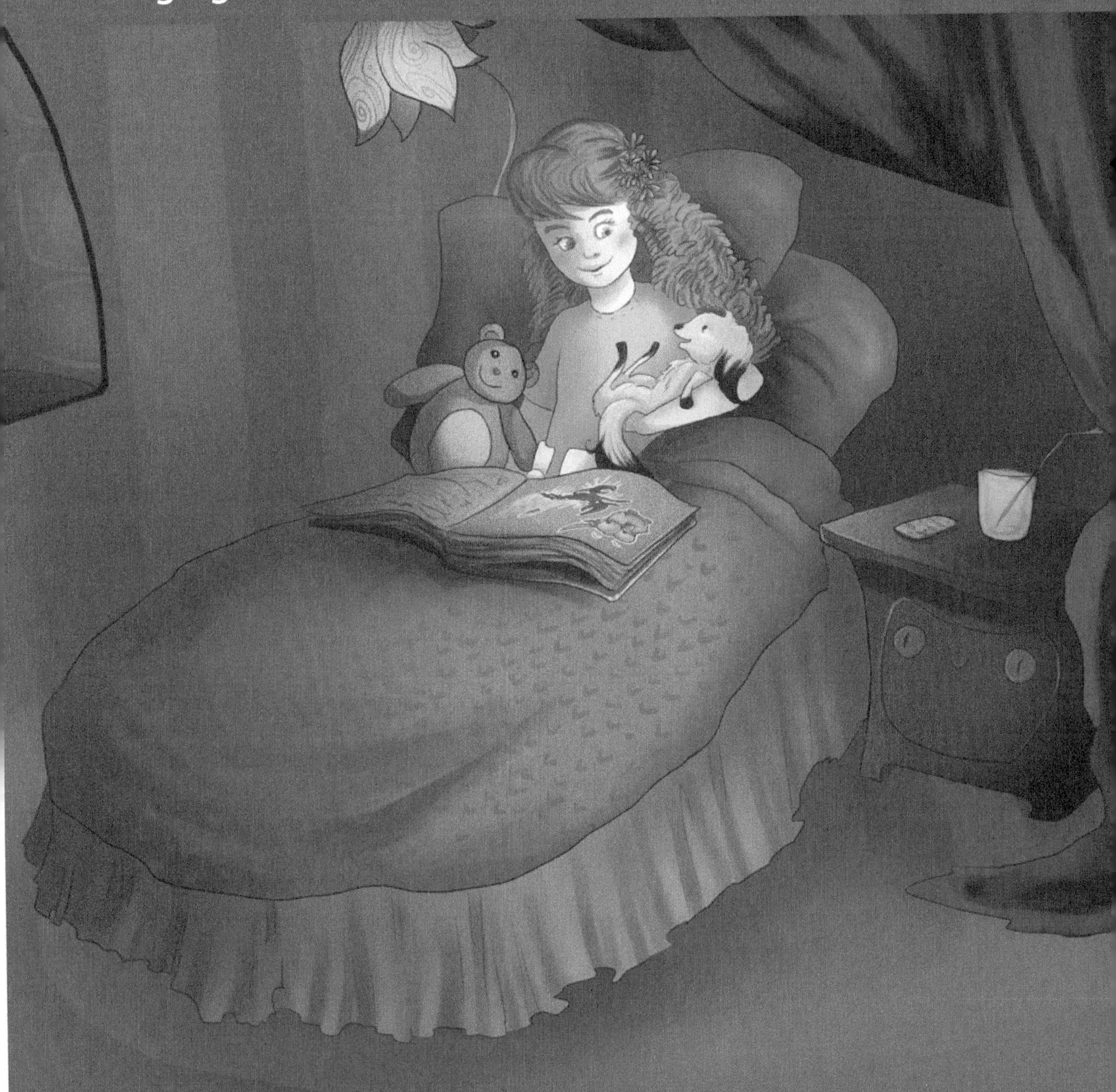

It is a nice day outside.

Dad says,
"Rosa, do you want
to go play outside?"

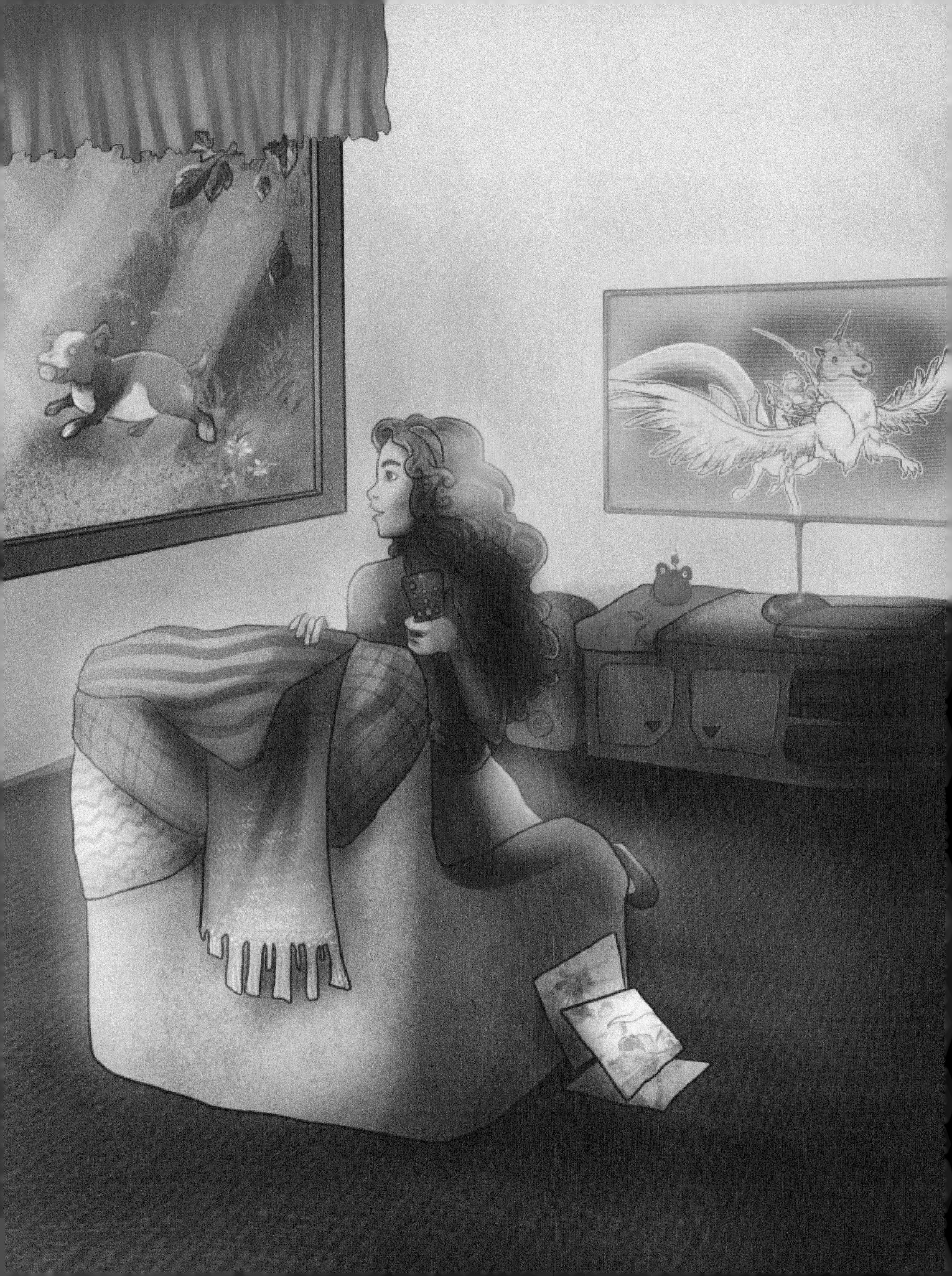

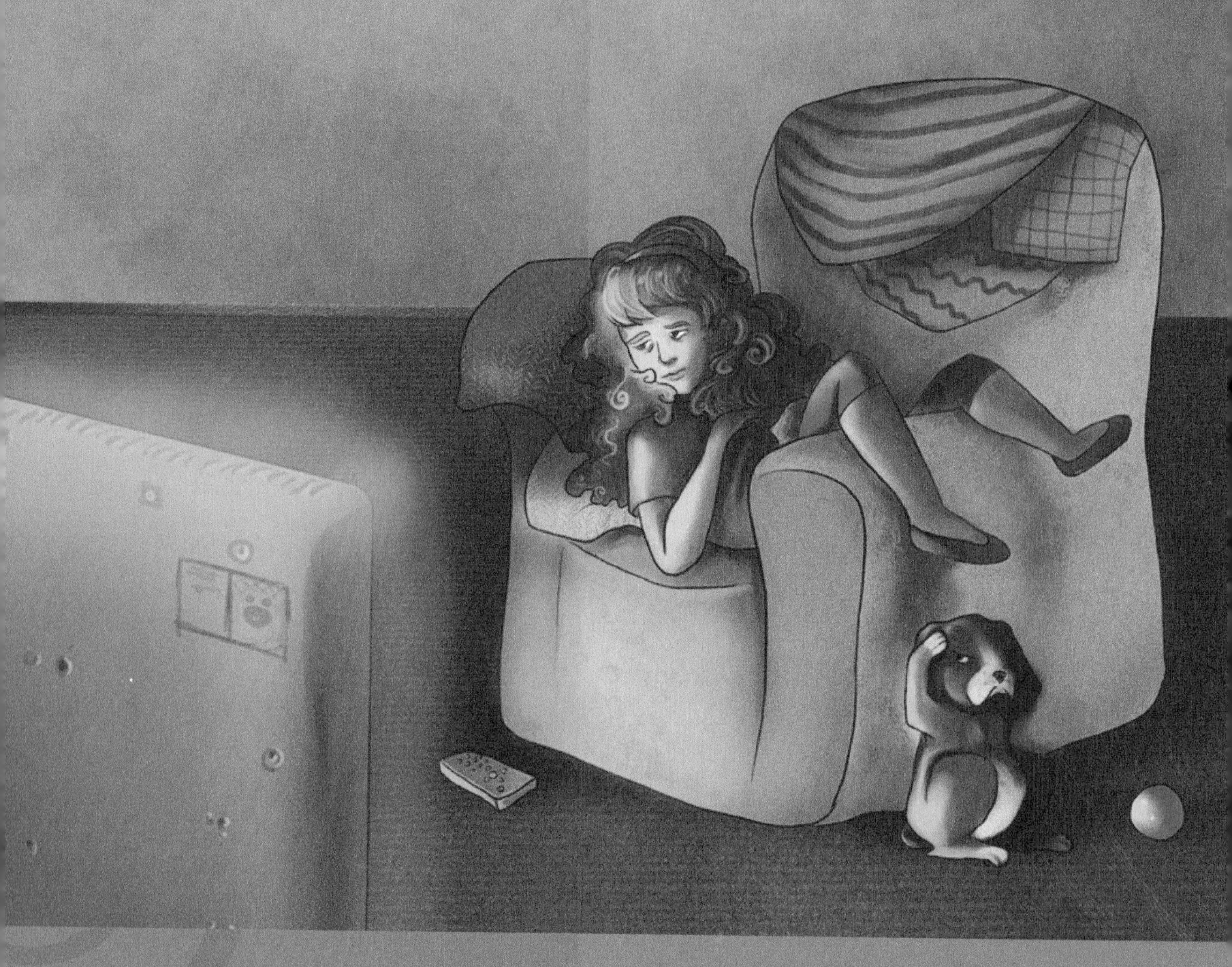

Rosa does not want to play outside.
She watches a movie. Her muscles feel droopy and weak.
She is not giving them the exercise they need
to grow strong and healthy.

Why is Rosa out of energy?

Rosa goes outside to play. She has fun running around and playing. Rosa's body gets the exercise it needs to be strong and healthy. She laughs as she jumps higher!

Rosa loves to play jump rope and hopscotch. What do you like to play outside?

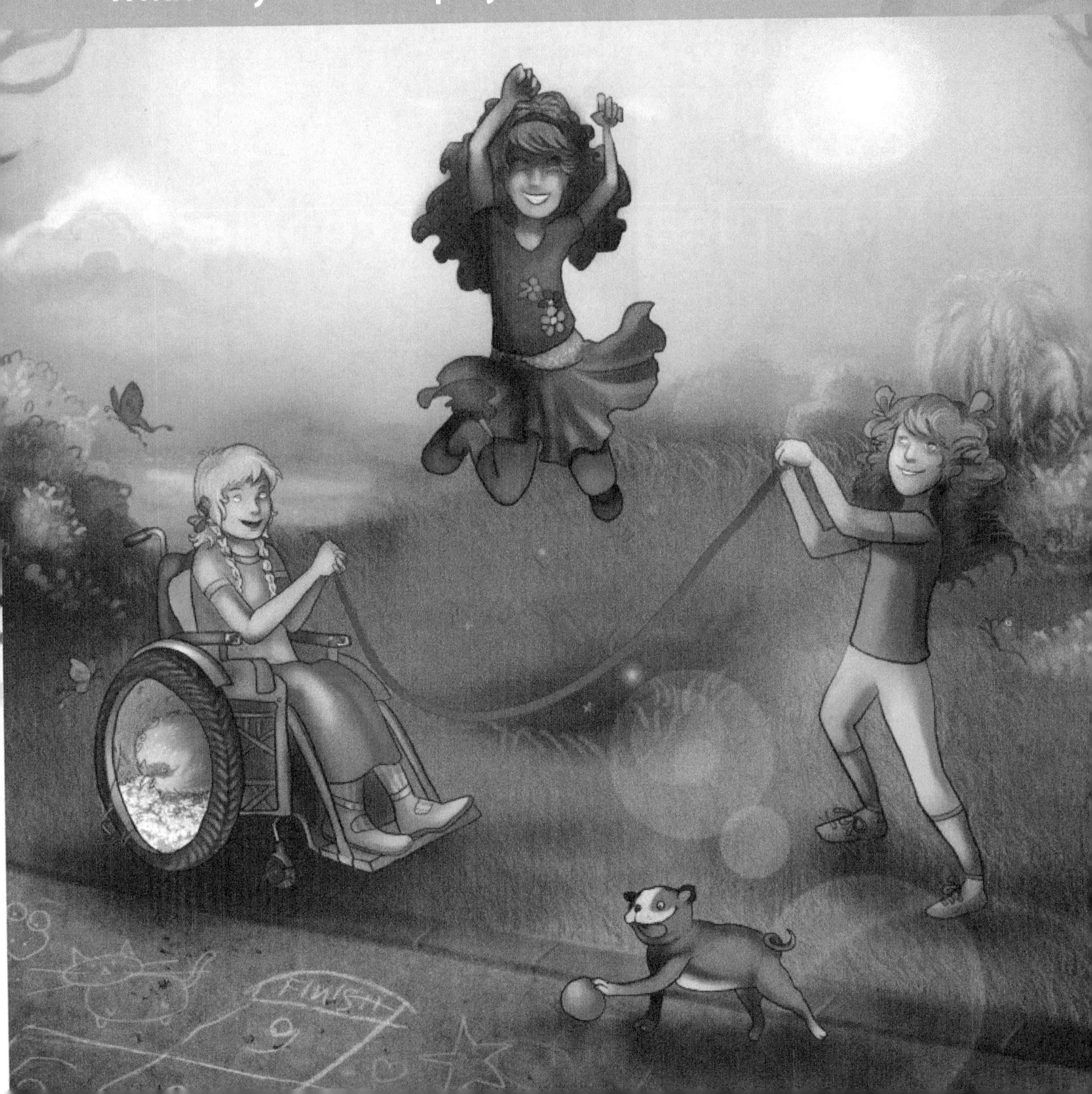

Jake is hungry.

He asks,
"May I please have a cookie?"

Mom says,
"You may have a cookie
after dinner. Feel free to have
a piece of fruit if you are
too hungry to wait."

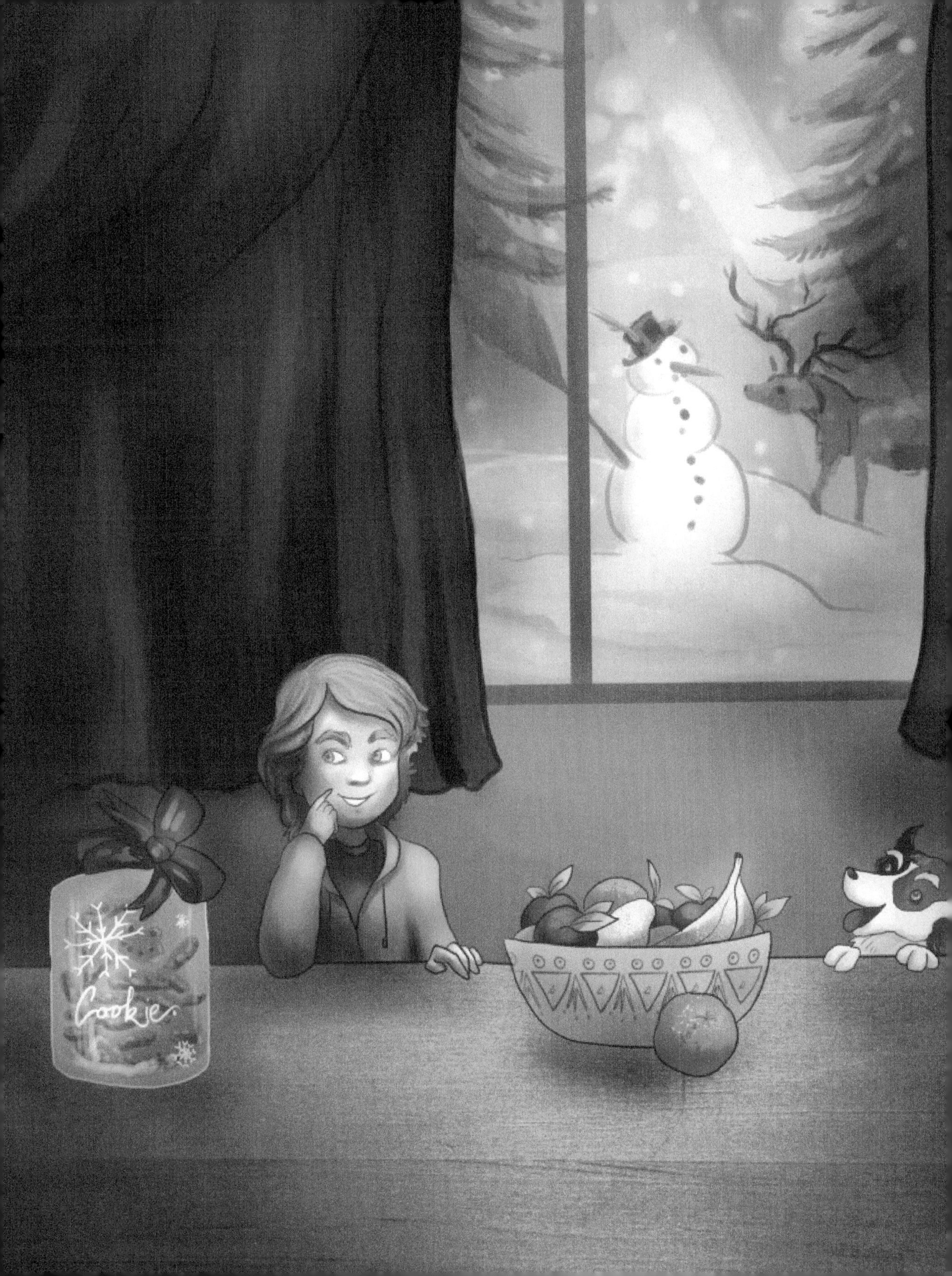
Cookie

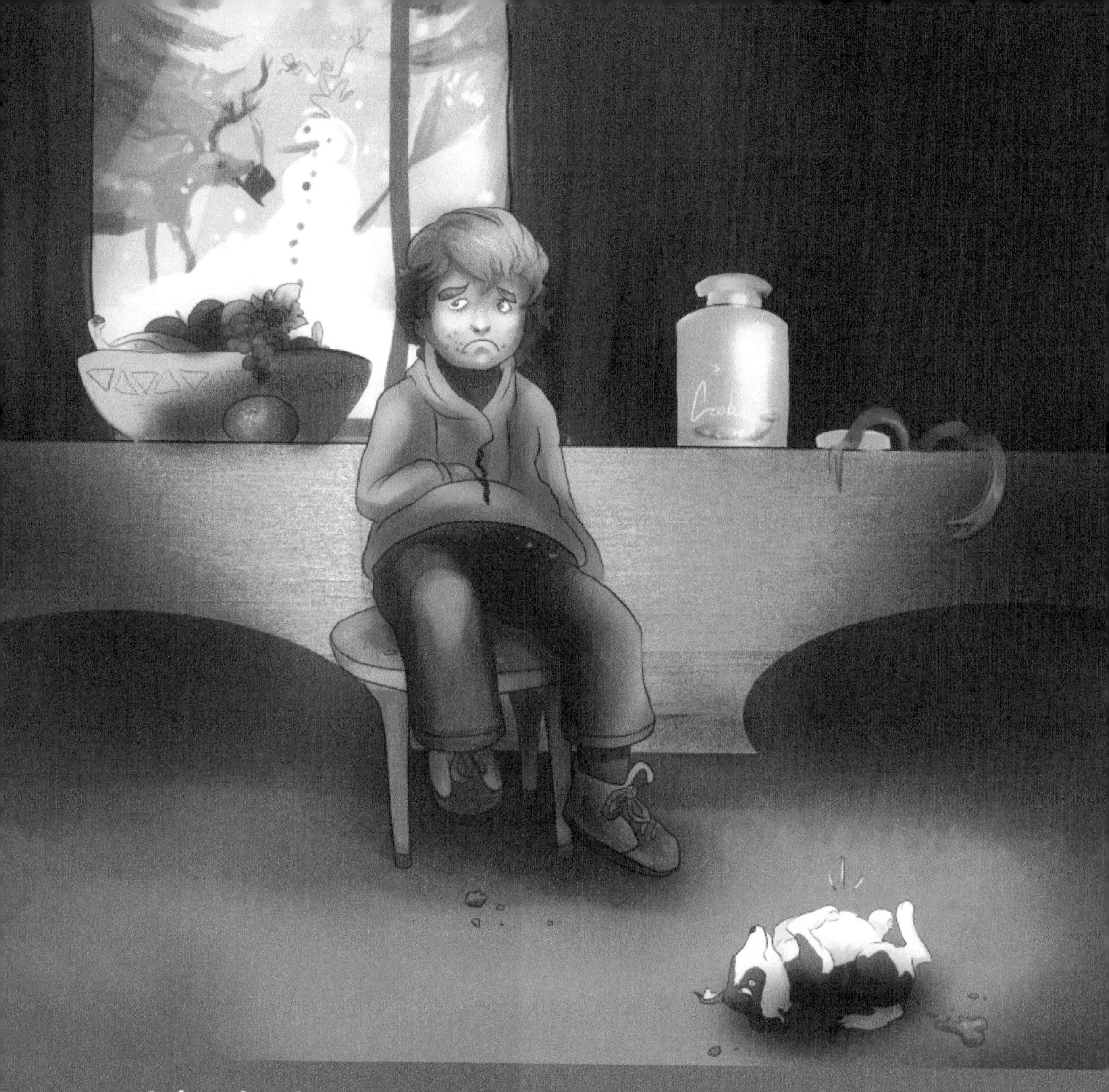

Jake thinks, "I do not want fruit. I want a cookie."
He eats three cookies!
Now, Jake does not have room in his tummy
for food that is good for his body.
Junk food will not keep Jake healthy and strong.

Why is Jake feeling bad?

Jake says, "Okay, Mom. What fruit do we have?"
Mom says, "We have apples, oranges, and grapes."
Jake says, "Yum! Can I have them all?"
Mom says, "What a good idea! Fruit salad is healthy and tasty."

Jake likes fruit for a healthy snack.
What is your favorite healthy snack?

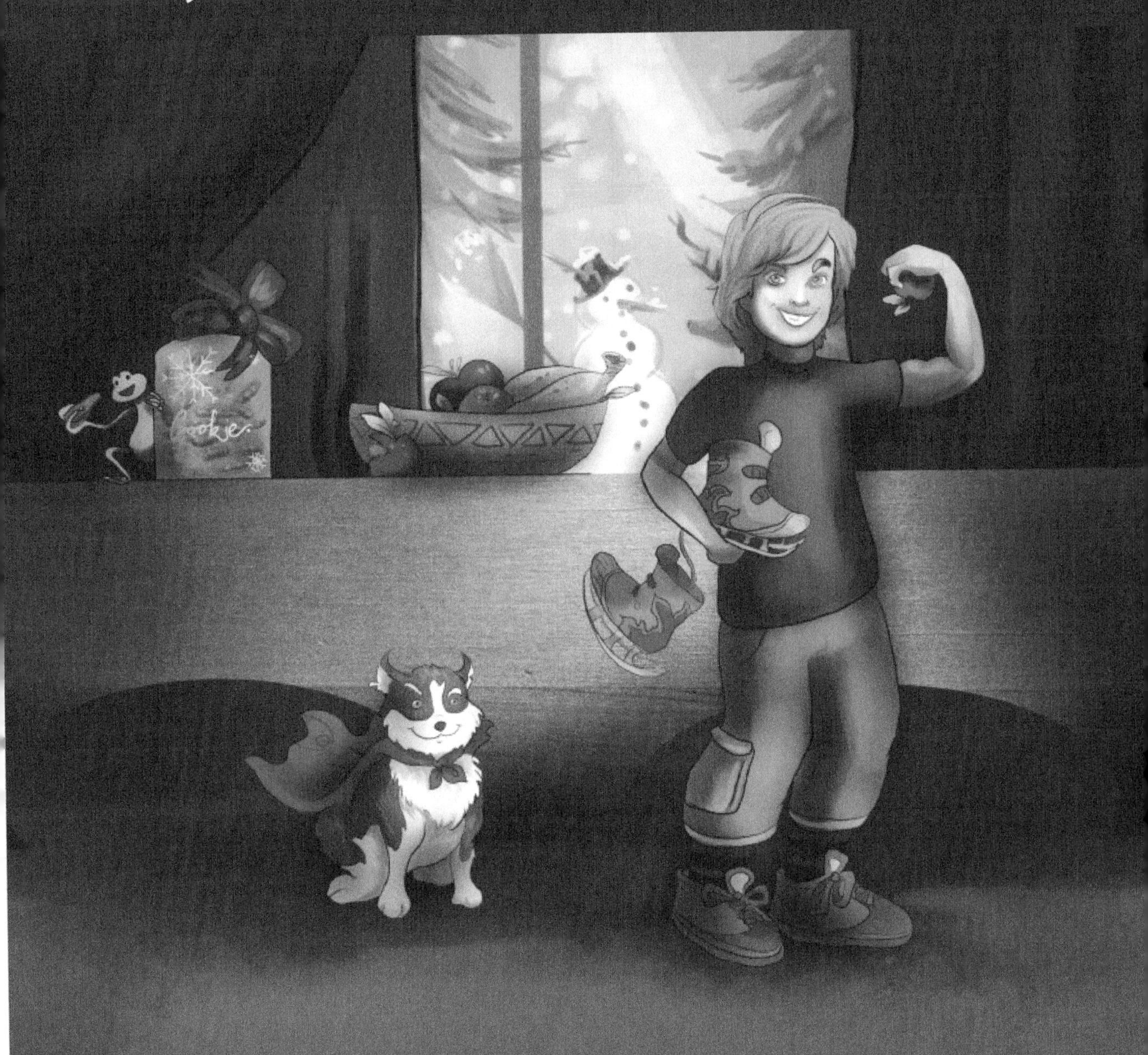

It is bedtime.

Dad says,
"Jalen, please turn
your light out.
It is time for bed."

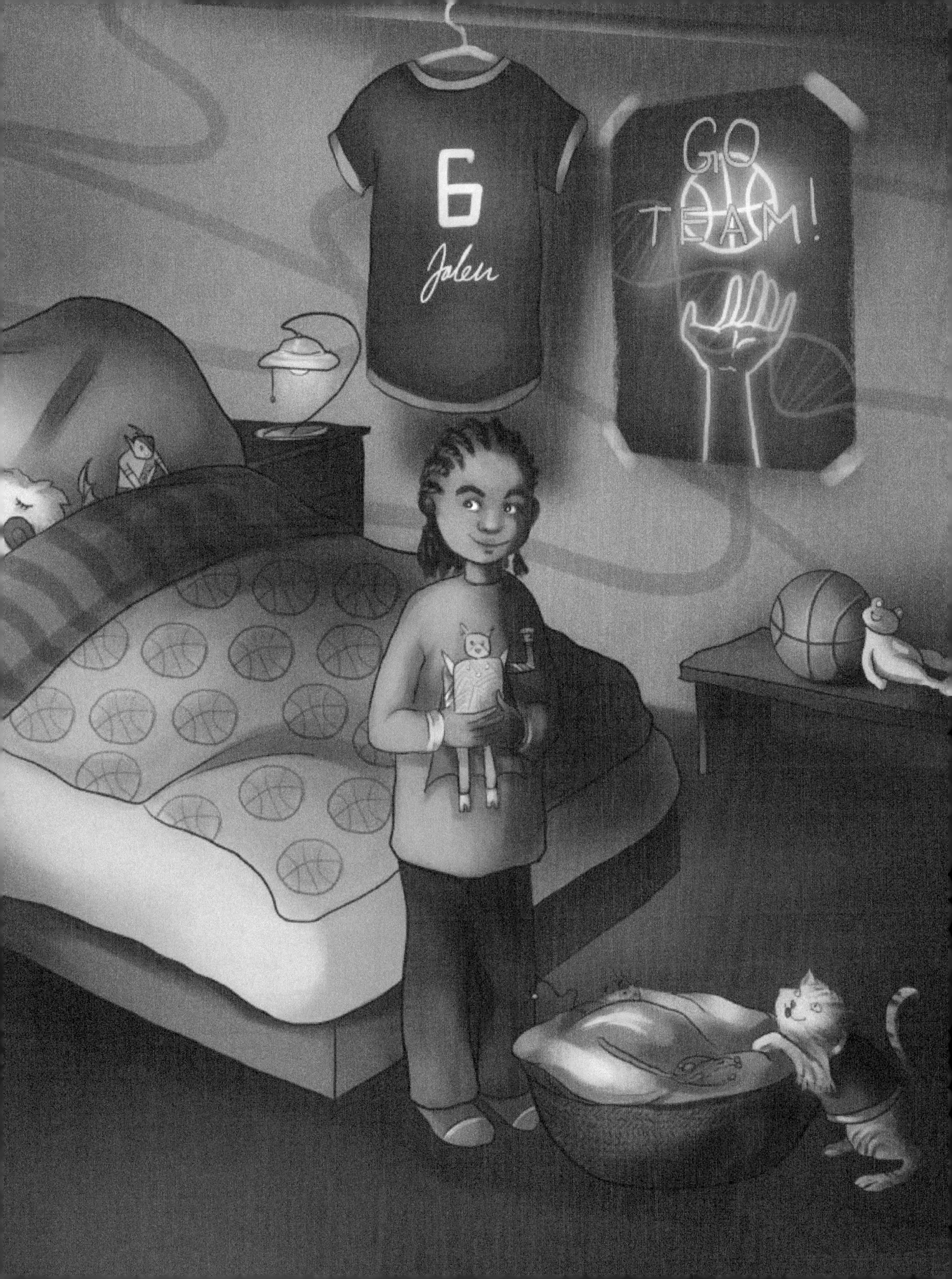
6
Jalen
GO
TEAM!

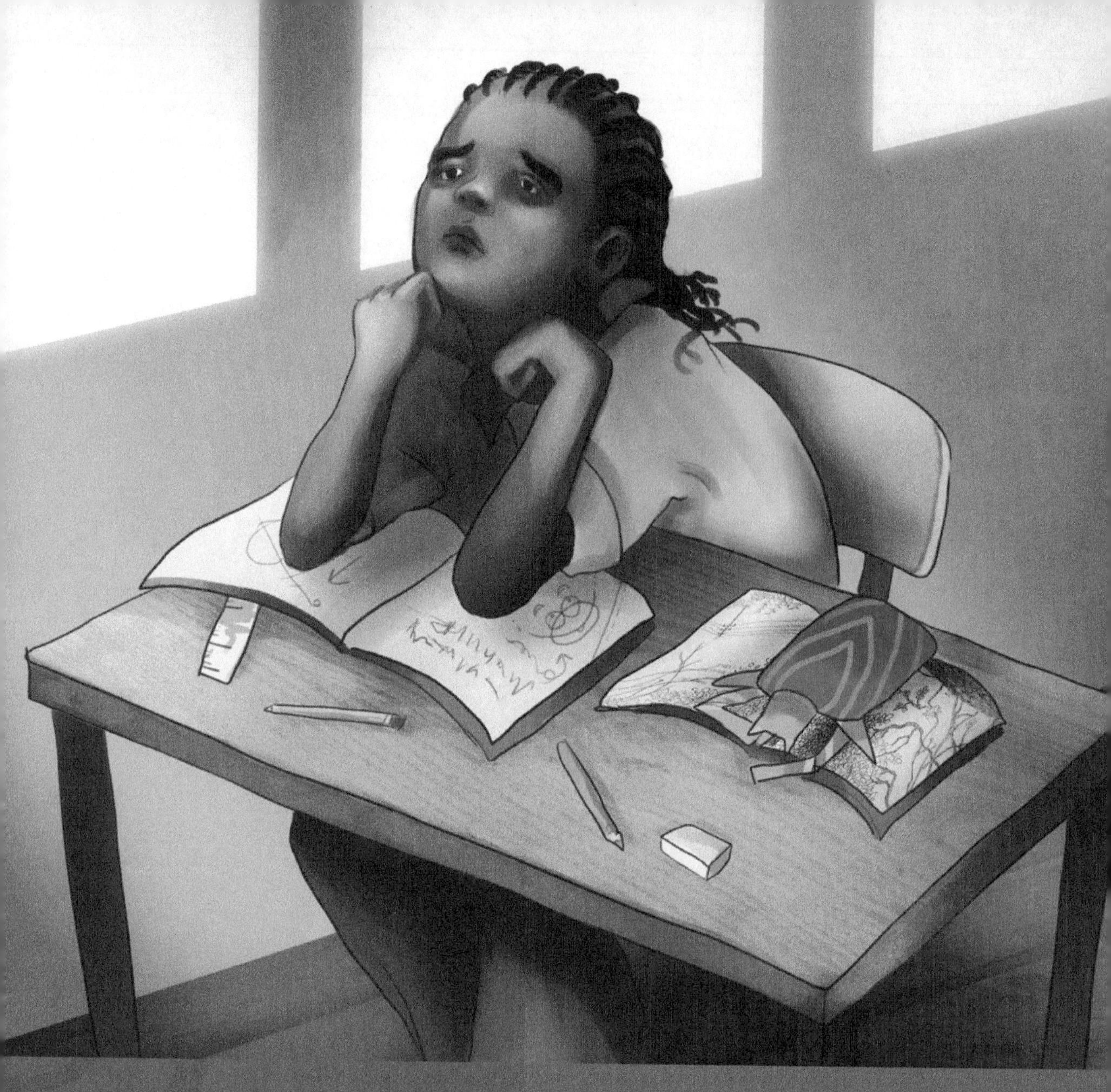

Jalen does not go to sleep at bedtime.
He stays up and plays with his toys.
Jalen feels sleepy in the morning.
He is too tired to learn or play at school.

Why is Jalen tired and grumpy?

Jalen goes to sleep at bedtime.
He feels good when he wakes up!
He is happy to go to school.
Jalen has lots of energy to learn and play with his friends.

Jalen likes math the best.
What do you like to learn at school?

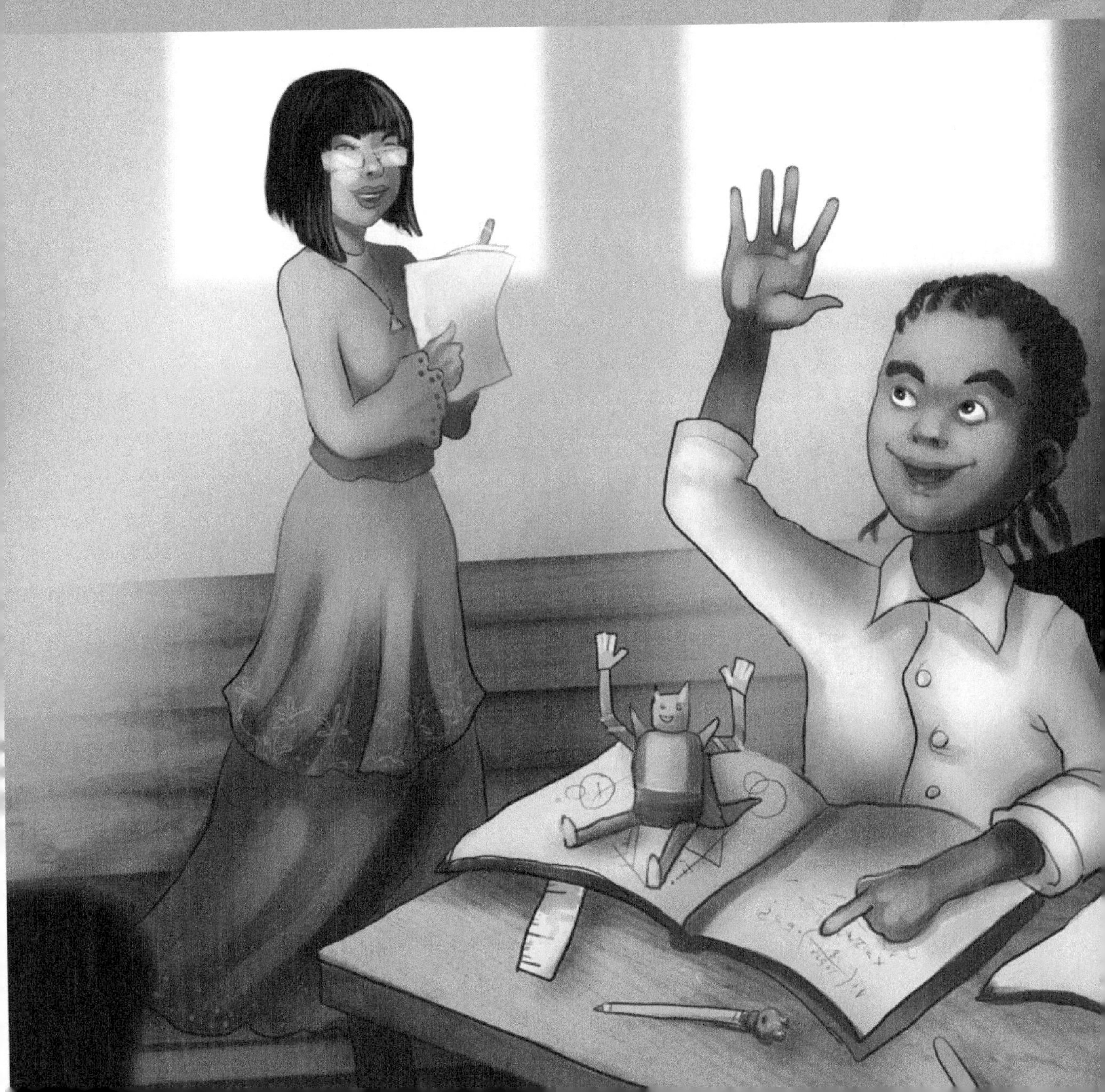

Kasey just came home
from school.

She is hungry.

Grandpa says,
"Kasey, please wash
your hands before
you eat a snack."

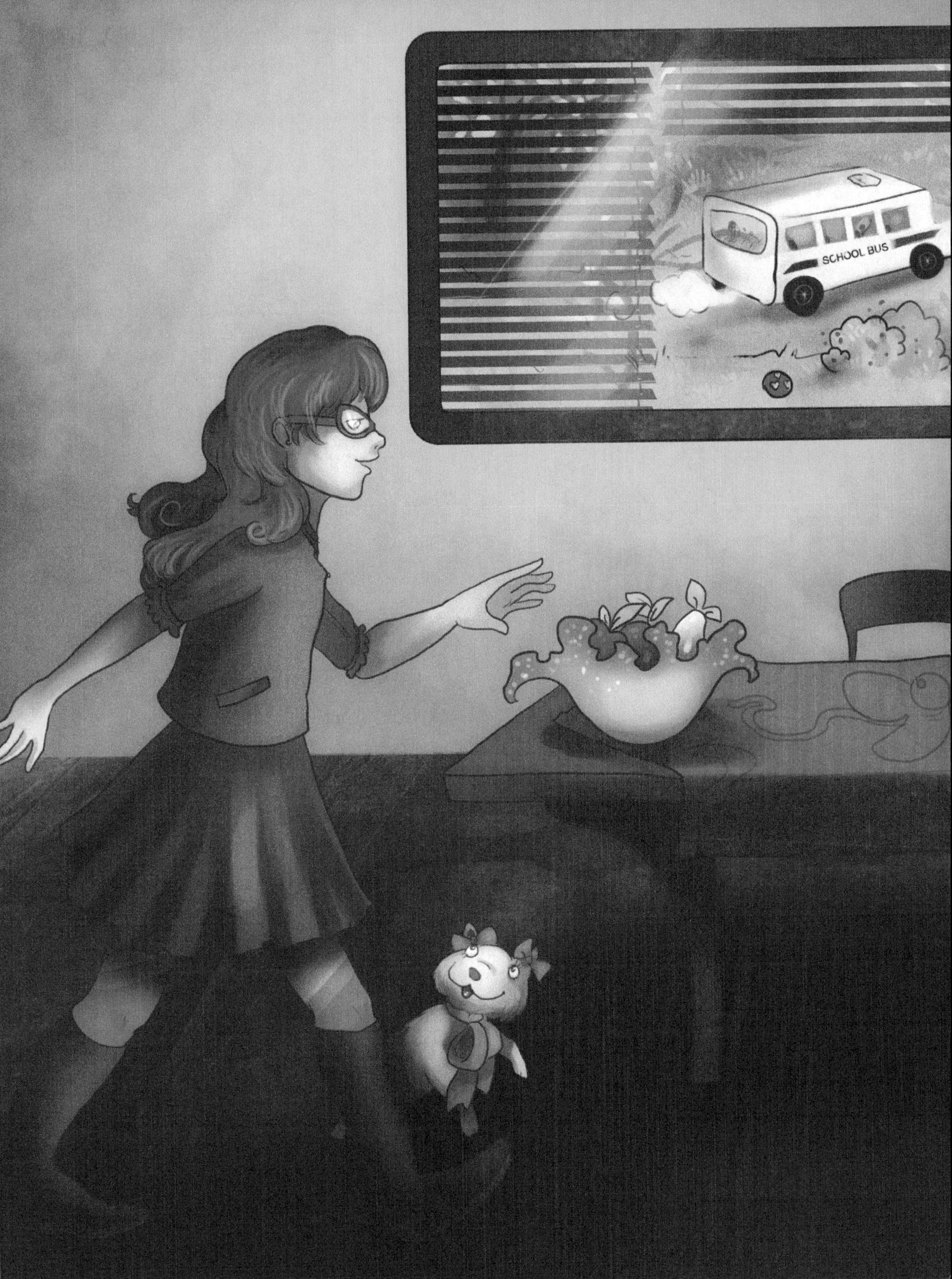
SCHOOL BUS

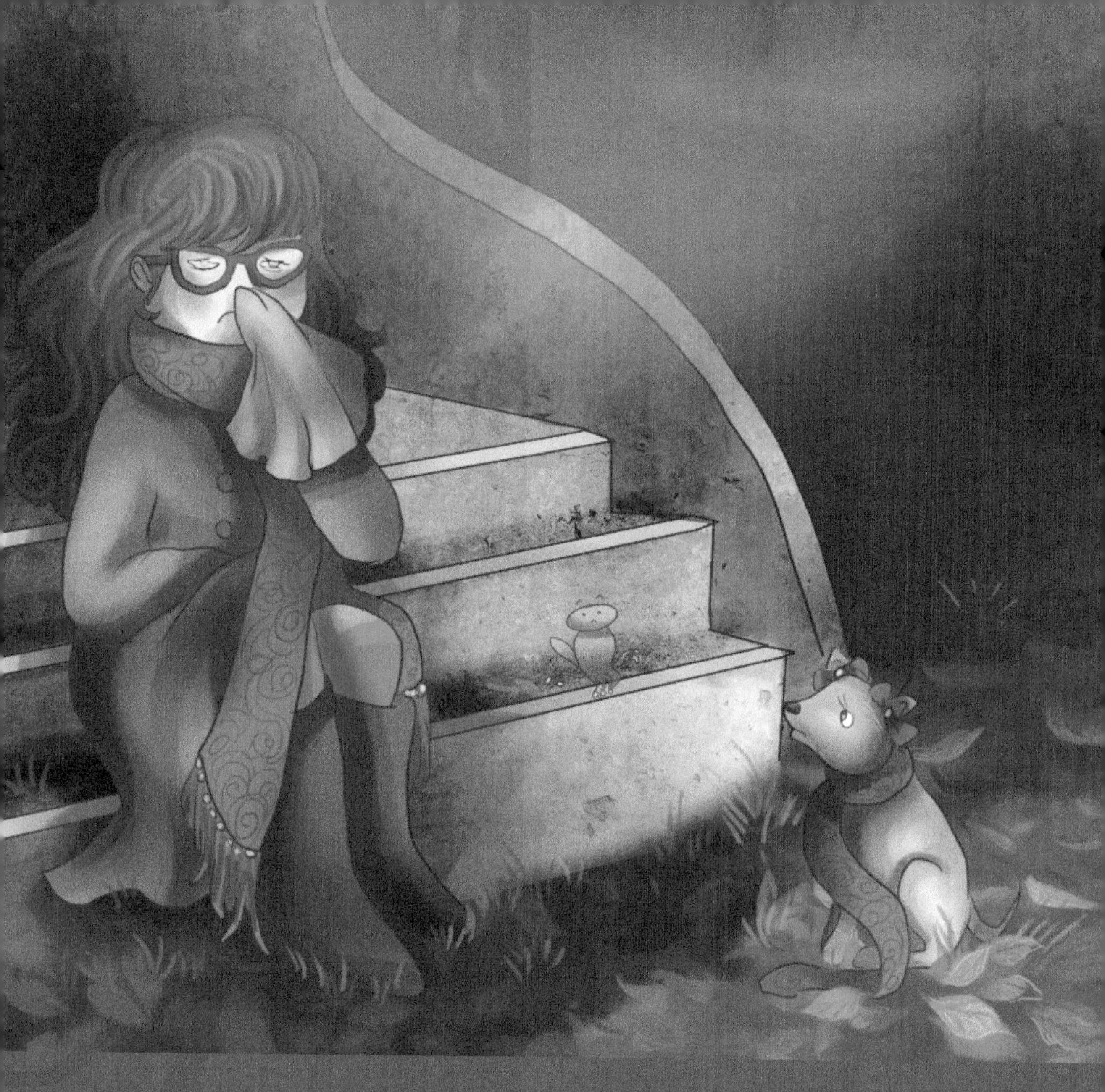

Kasey did not wash her hands.
Her hands had bad germs on them.
They gave her a cold. Now, Kasey is sick.
She is sad that she feels too sick to play.

Why is Kasey not feeling well?

Kasey washes her hands. The soap and water kills bad germs that can make her sick.
Kasey is happy that the germs are gone.
They will not make her sick. Now she can play!

Kasey likes to play with her ball.
What games do you like to play?

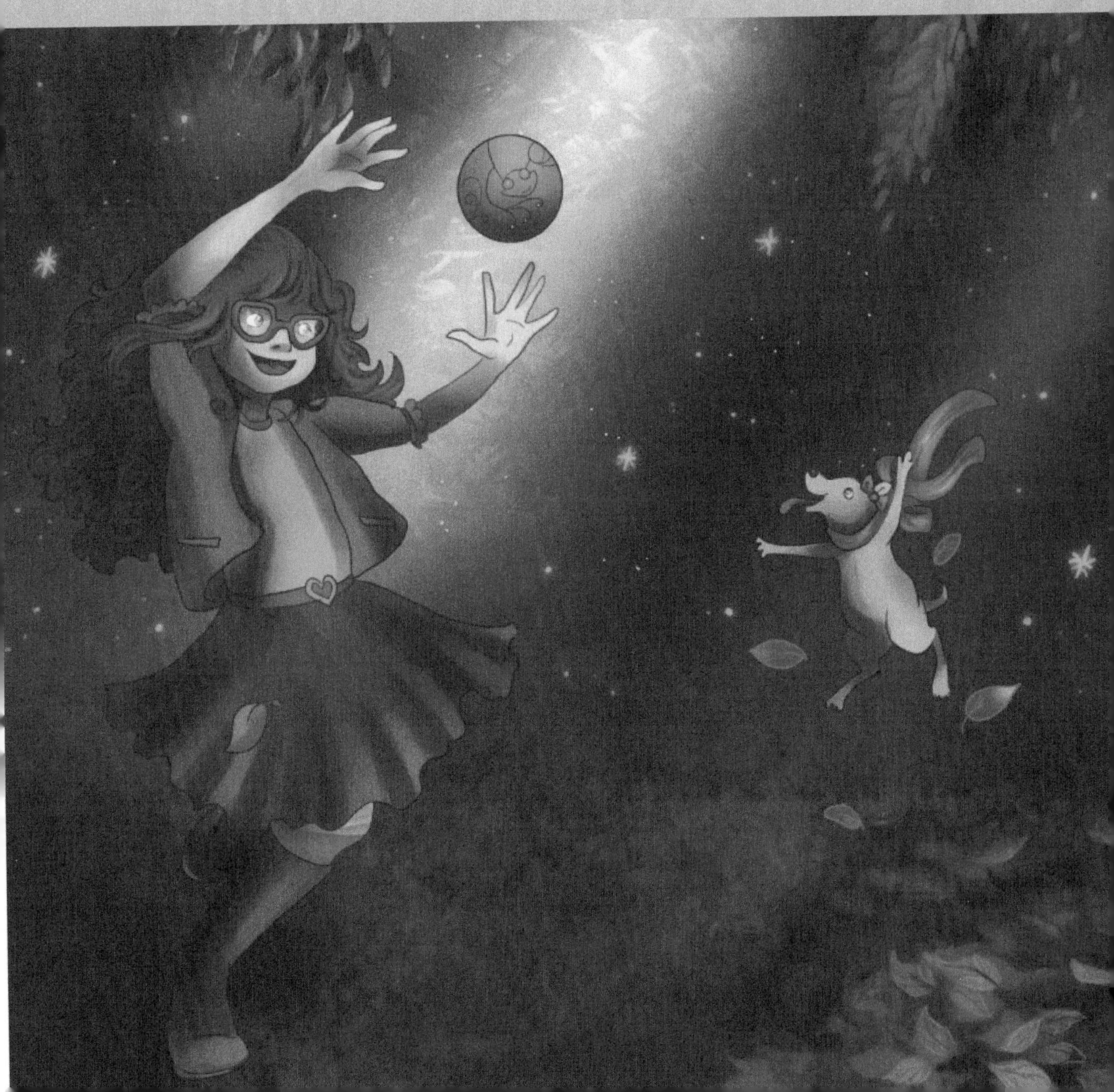

Aydin is at the doctor's office
for a check-up.

Mom says,
"Aydin, the nurse is ready
to give you a vaccine.
It will help your body
stay healthy.
Which arm would you
like it in?"

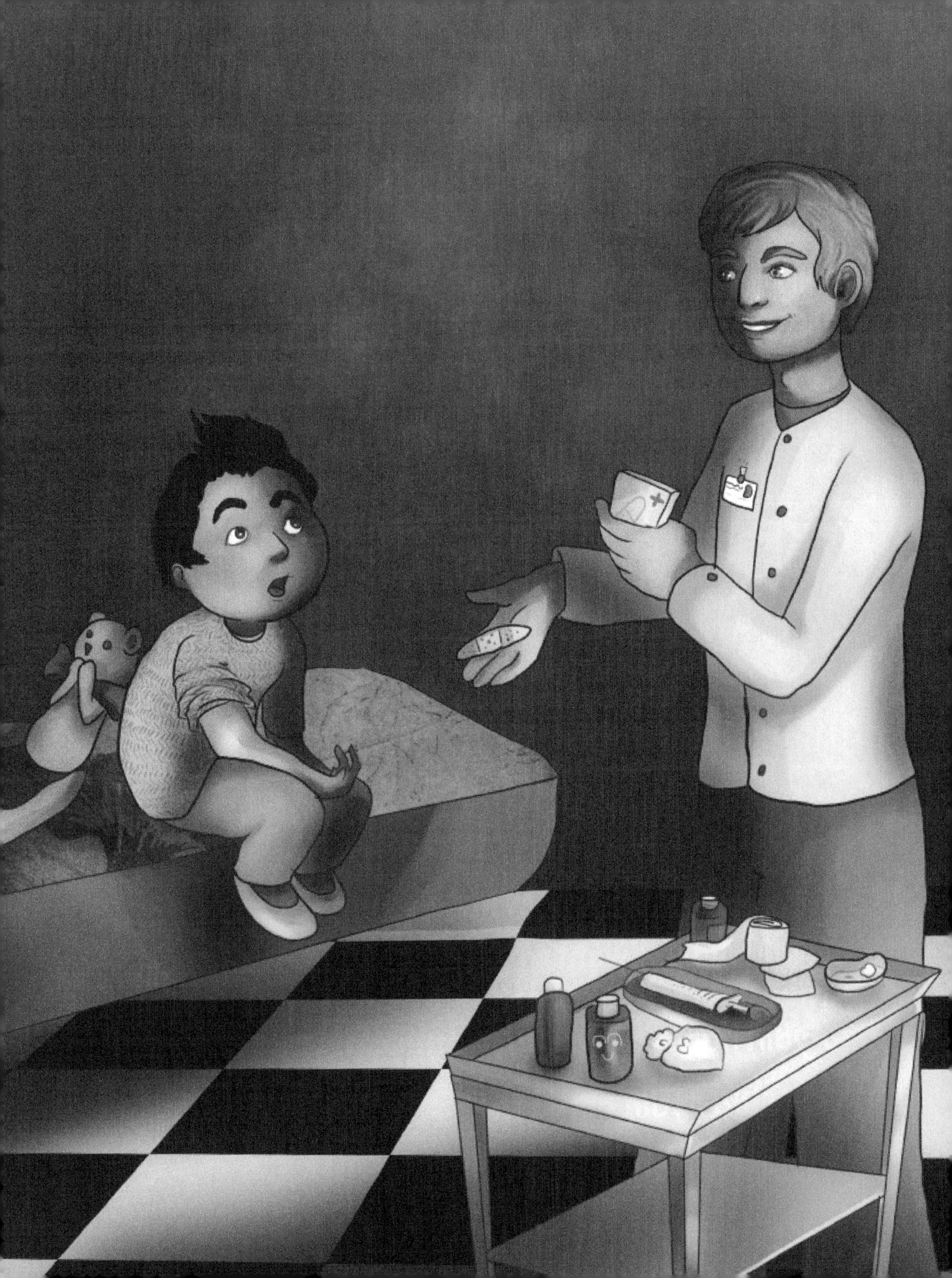

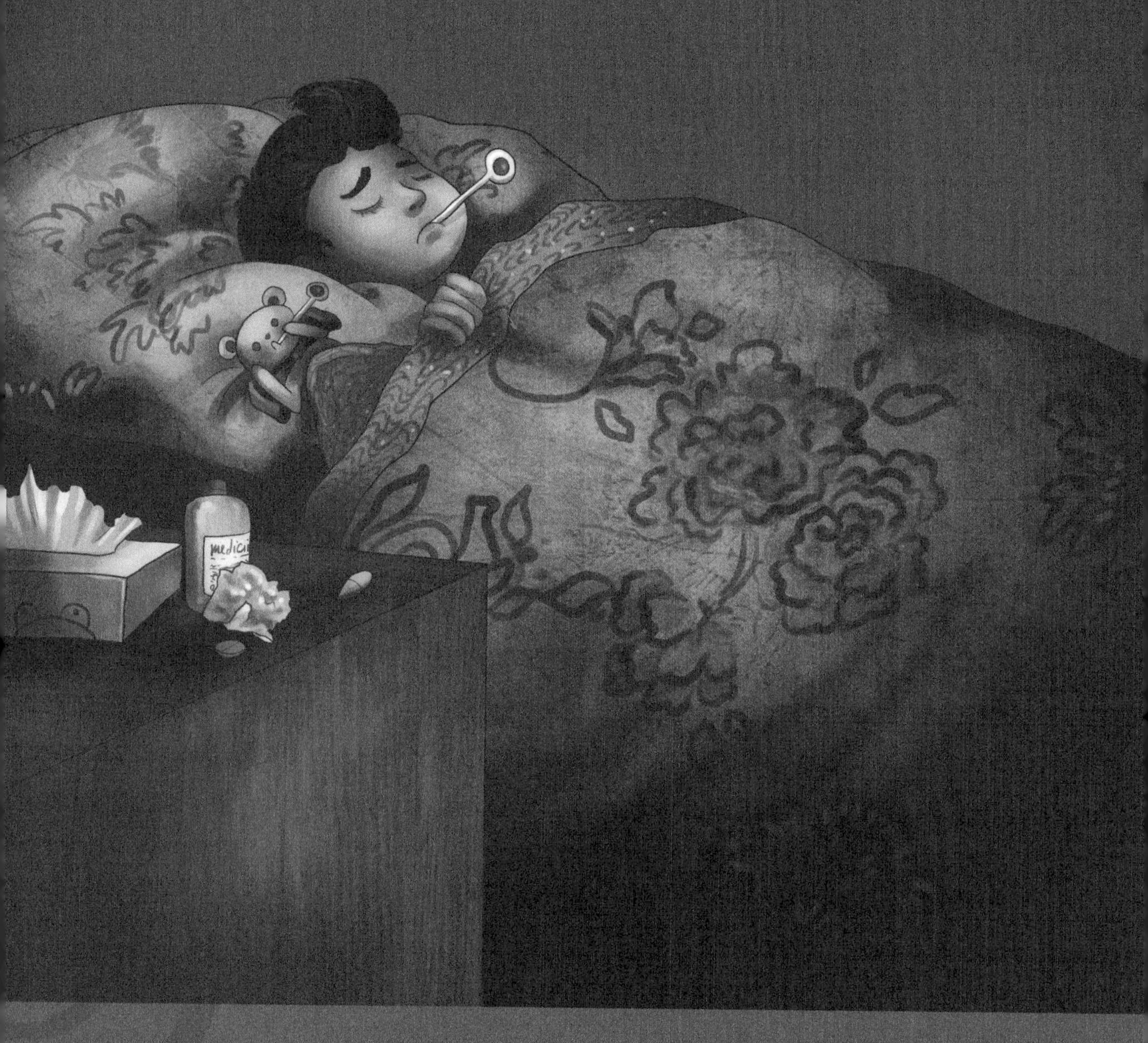

Aydin did not want to get a poke in his arm.
Now he is sick and has to stay in bed.
Aydin hopes he will feel better soon.

Why did Aydin get sick?

Aydin lets the nurse give him a shot. He is very brave.
He holds still, turns his head and shuts his eyes.
It is very fast! Nurse gives him a superhero bandage.
Aydin says, "That was not so bad. Now I can stay healthy!"

Aydin likes to get a milkshake after his check-up.
What do you like to do?

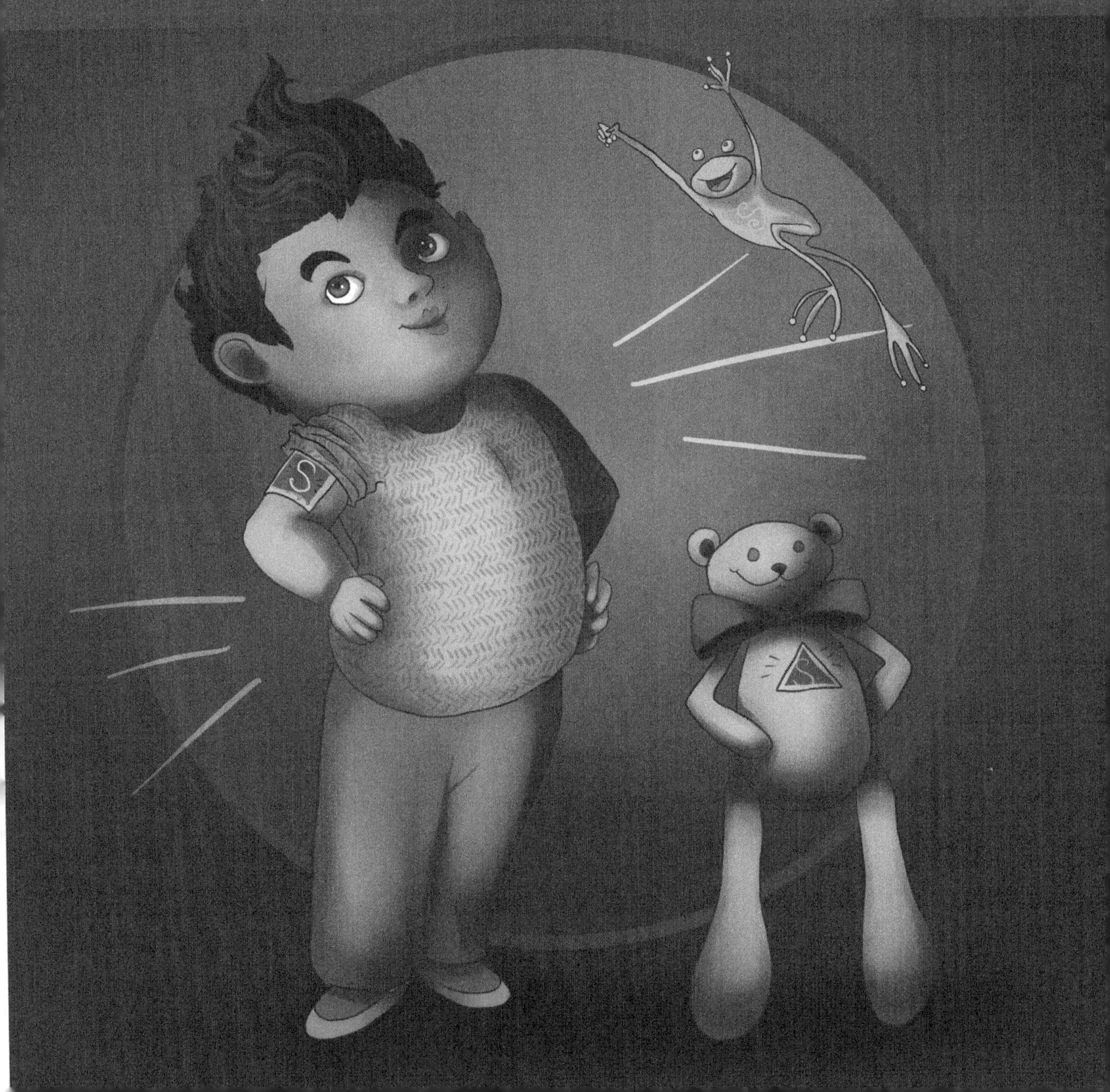

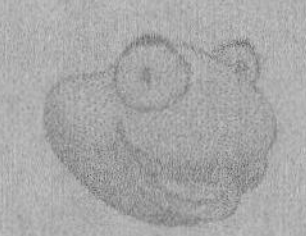

Maddie feels sick.

She goes to the doctor.

Doctor asks,
"Maddie, where does it hurt?"

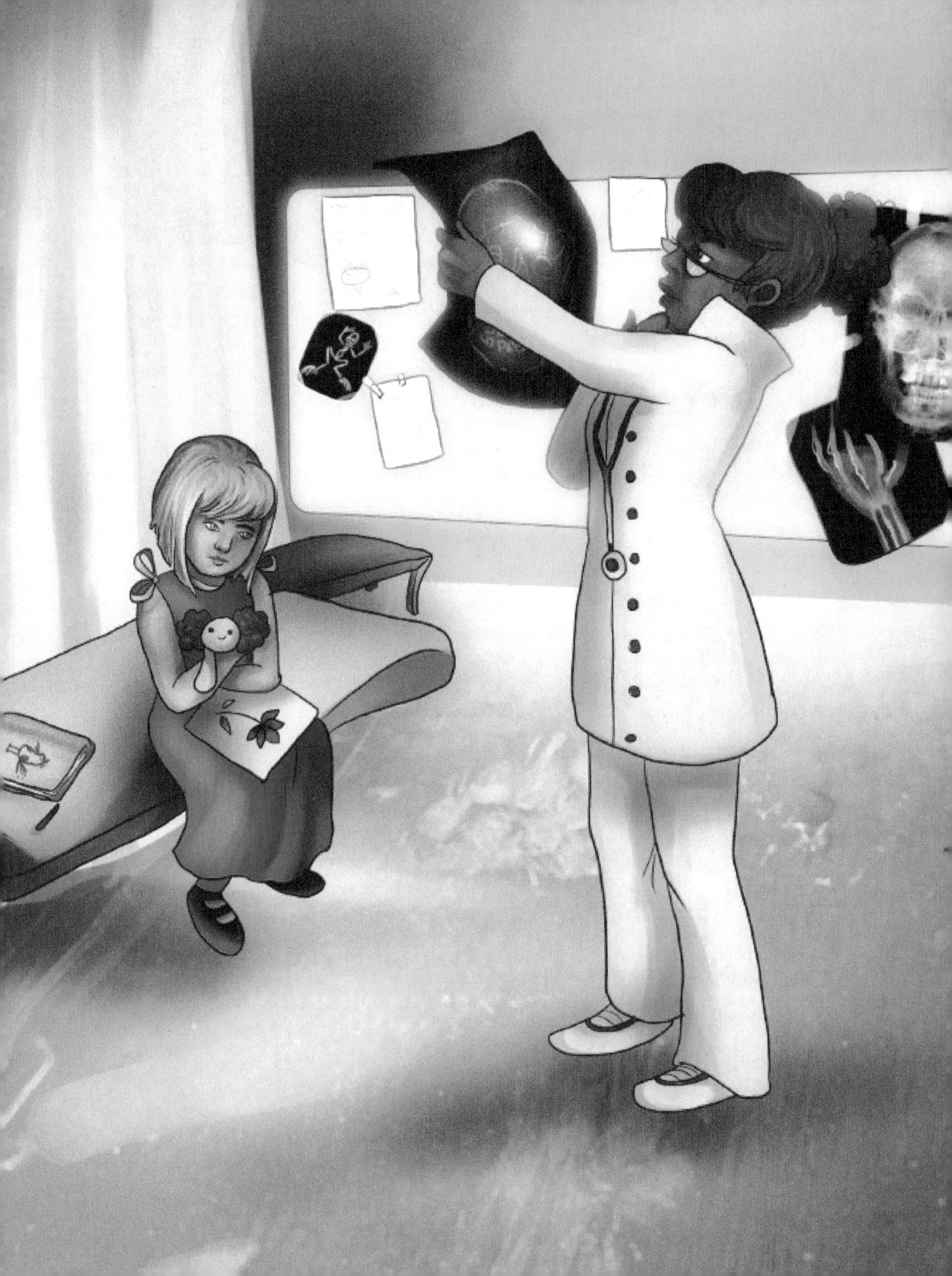

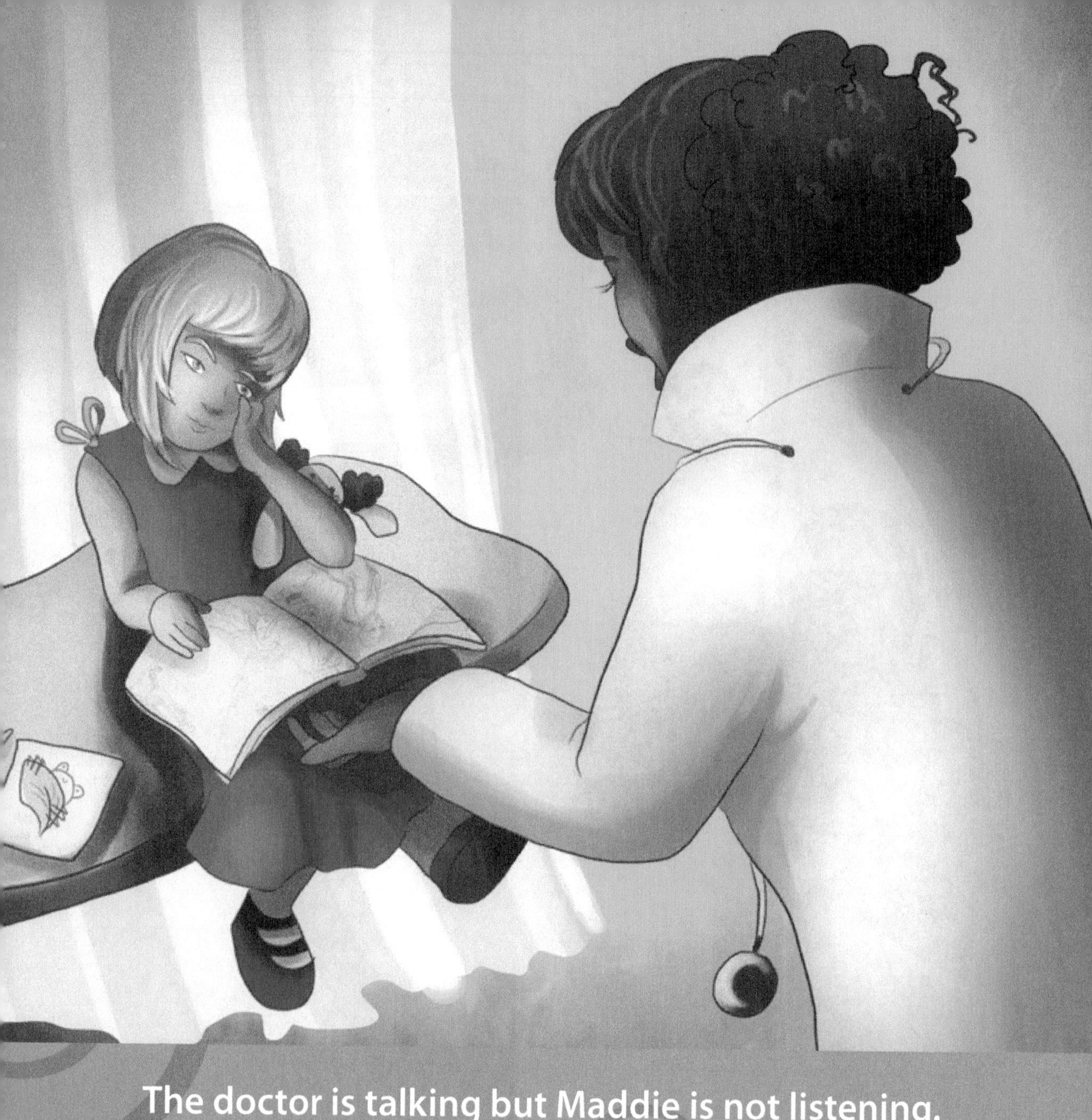

The doctor is talking but Maddie is not listening.
Doctor says, "Maddie, if you do what I say,
you will feel better."
Maddie does not know what
the doctor told her to do.

Why is Maddie sad?

Maddie sits still and listens to the doctor.
Doctor tells her what to do to feel better.
Maddie is proud of herself for listening.

Maddie likes to learn how to take good care of her body.
What do you like to learn about?

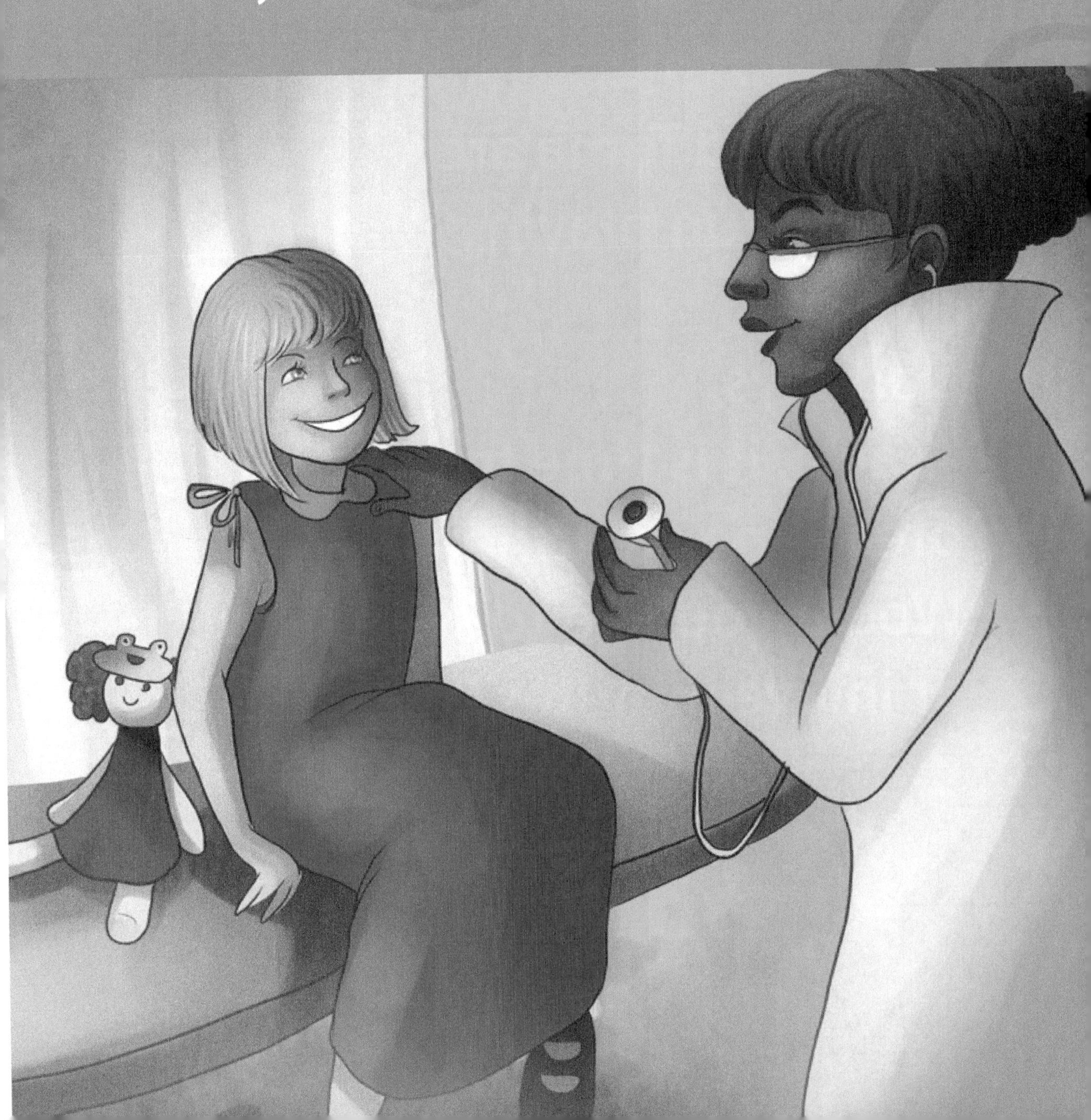

Kayla and Tama are
having fun playing.

Dad says,
“Kayla, it is time for your
breathing treatment.
Would you like to start now
or in five minutes?”

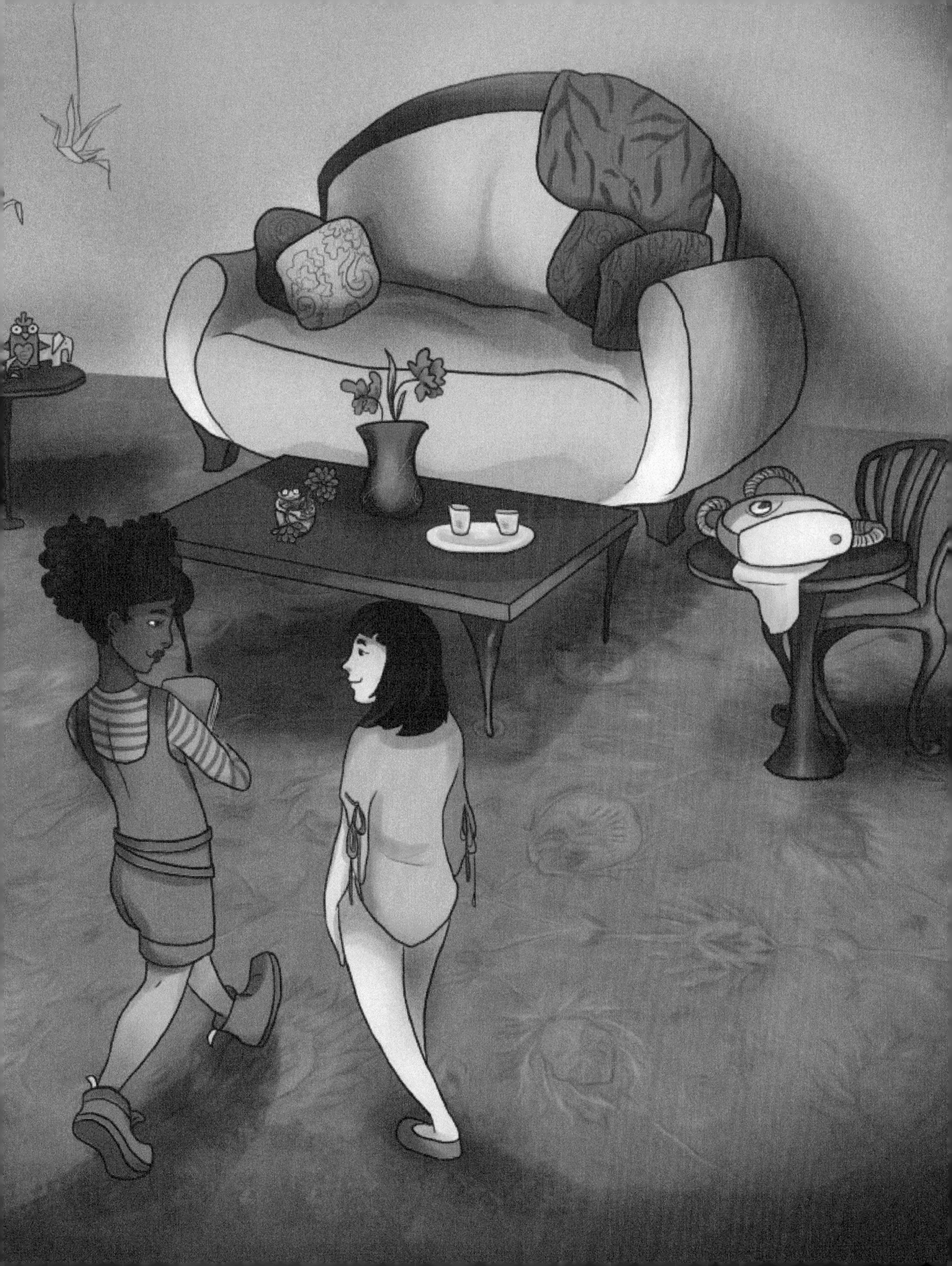

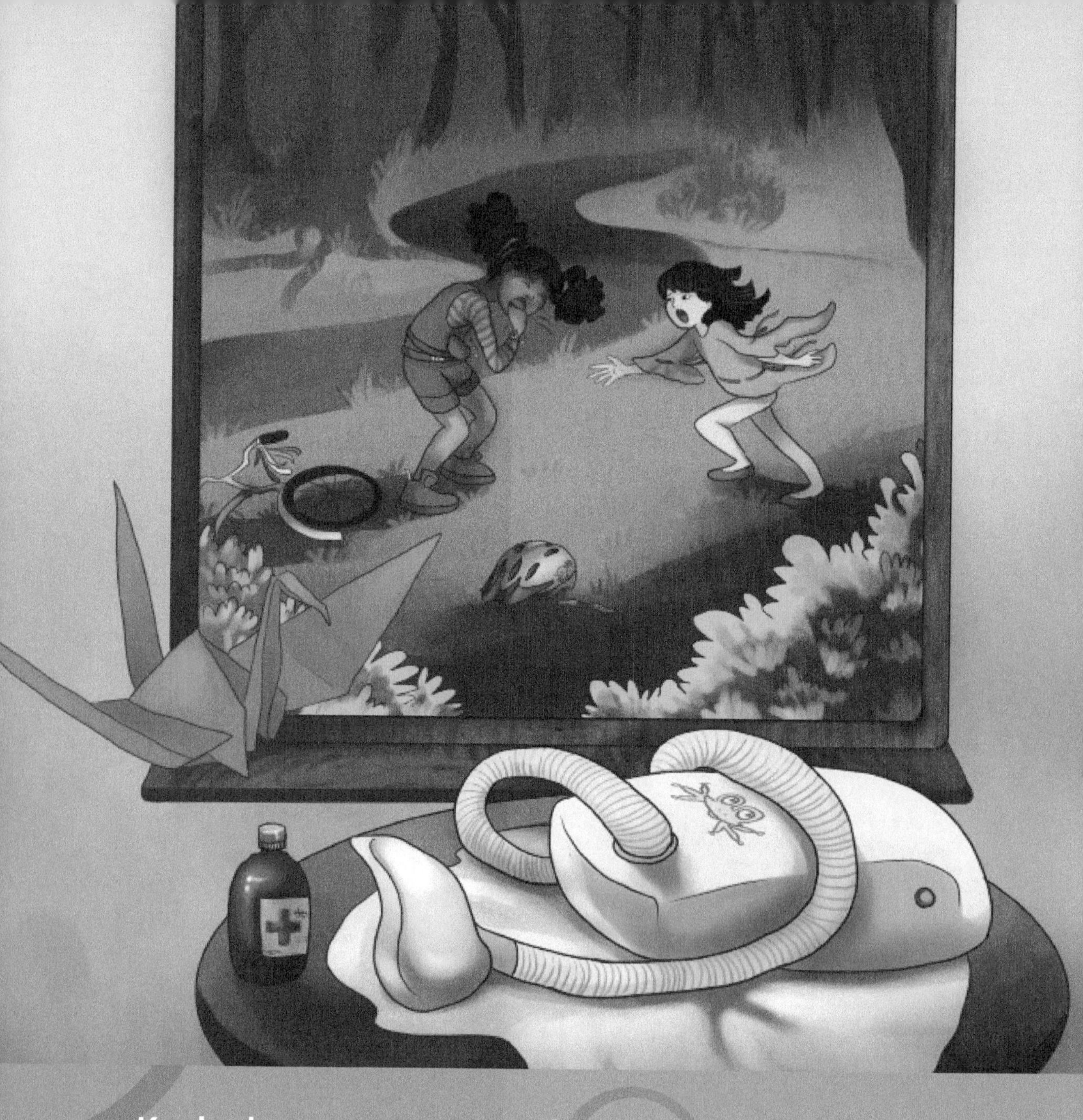

Kayla does not want to take her medicine.
She goes outside with Tama to ride bikes.
Kayla starts coughing.

Why is Kayla having a hard time breathing?

Kayla does her breathing treatment.
Kayla and Tama play a game
while the medicine goes into Kayla's lungs.

What other fun things could they do while
Kayla takes her medicine?

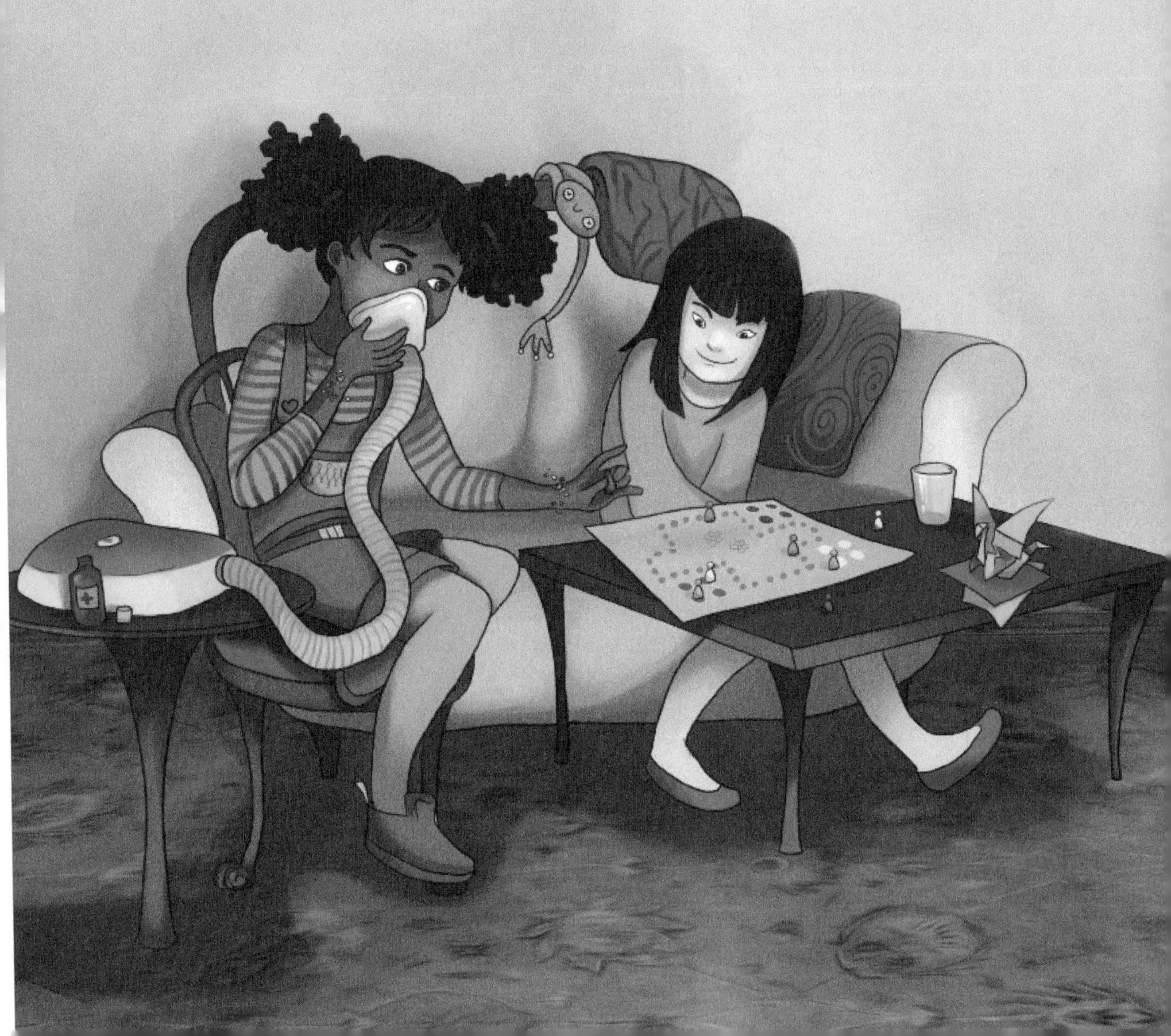

Mom says,
"Elliott, we should go to
the dentist so he can look
at your hurt tooth."

Elliott says,
"My tooth is fine.
I do not want to go
to the dentist.
I want to go to the beach!"

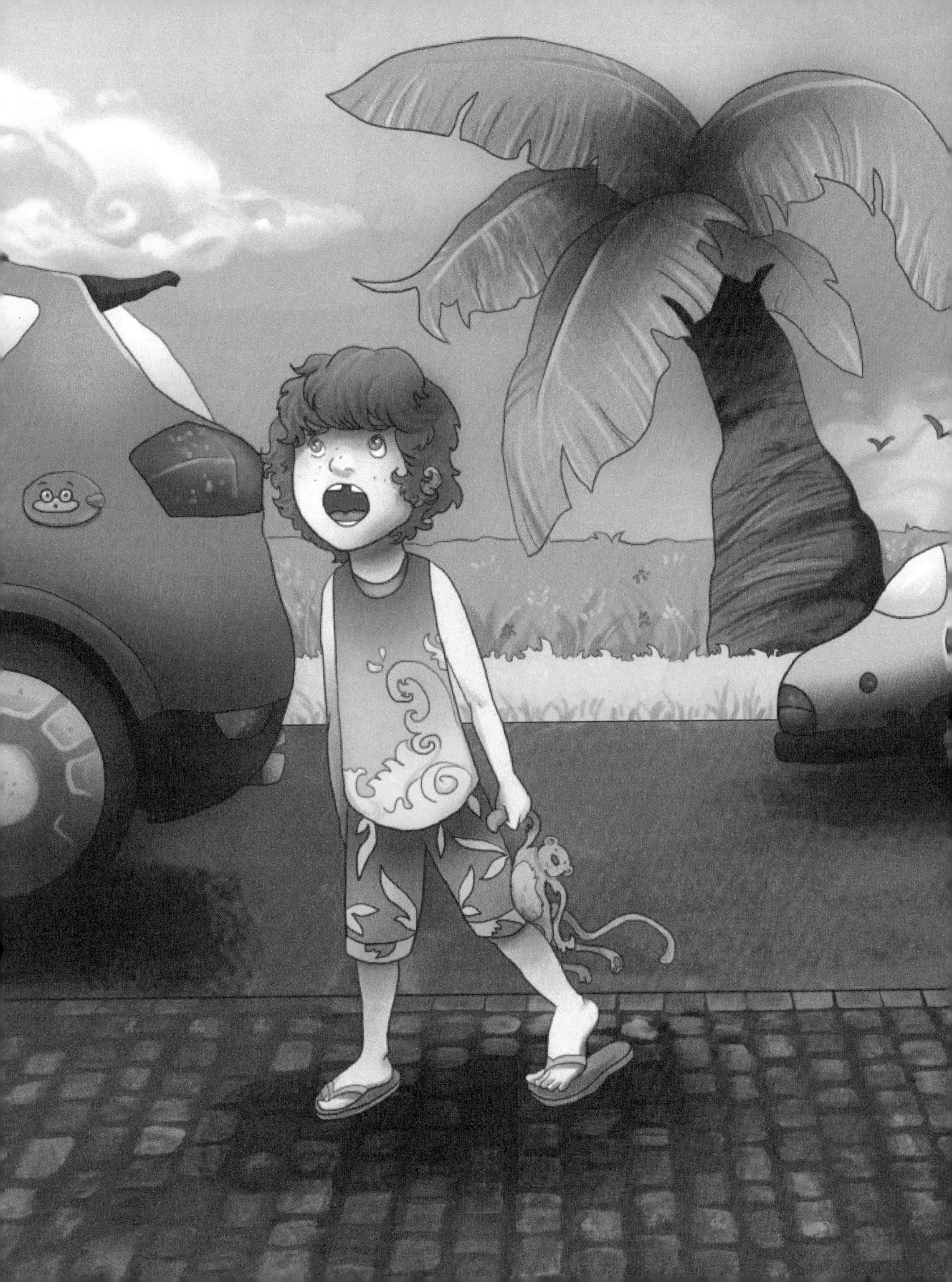

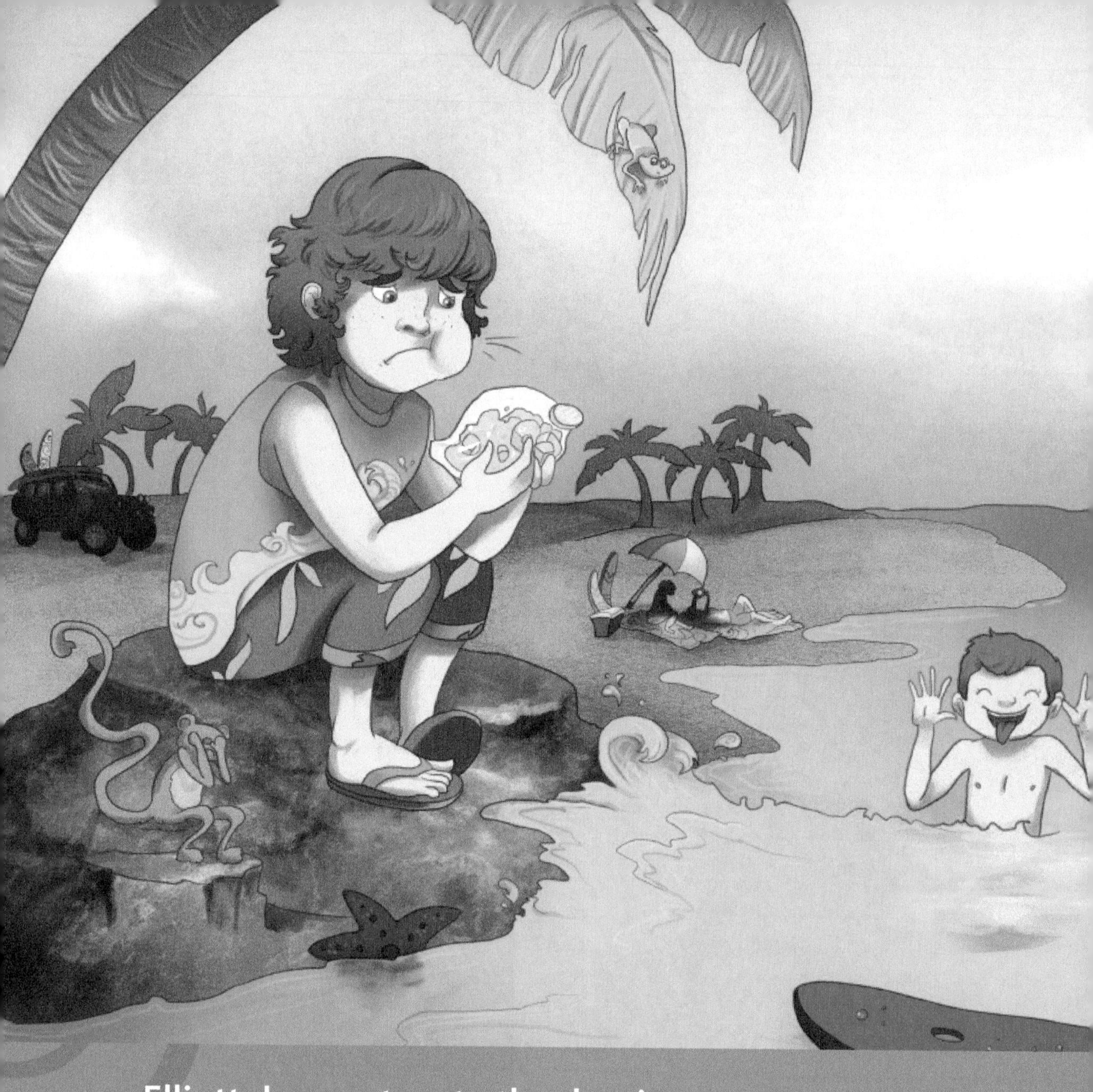

Elliott does not go to the dentist.
Later, Elliott cries, “Mom! My tooth hurts so bad!”
Mom says, “I am sorry your tooth hurts.
You may have a cavity.
This is why it is good to go to the dentist.”

Why does Elliott wish he had gone to the dentist?

Elliott gets his tooth checked by the dentist.
Dentist says, "Good job, Elliott. We fixed your cavity.
Be sure to brush your teeth twice a day,
limit sweets, and floss every day."

Elliott likes bubble gum flavored toothpaste.
What flavor do you like?

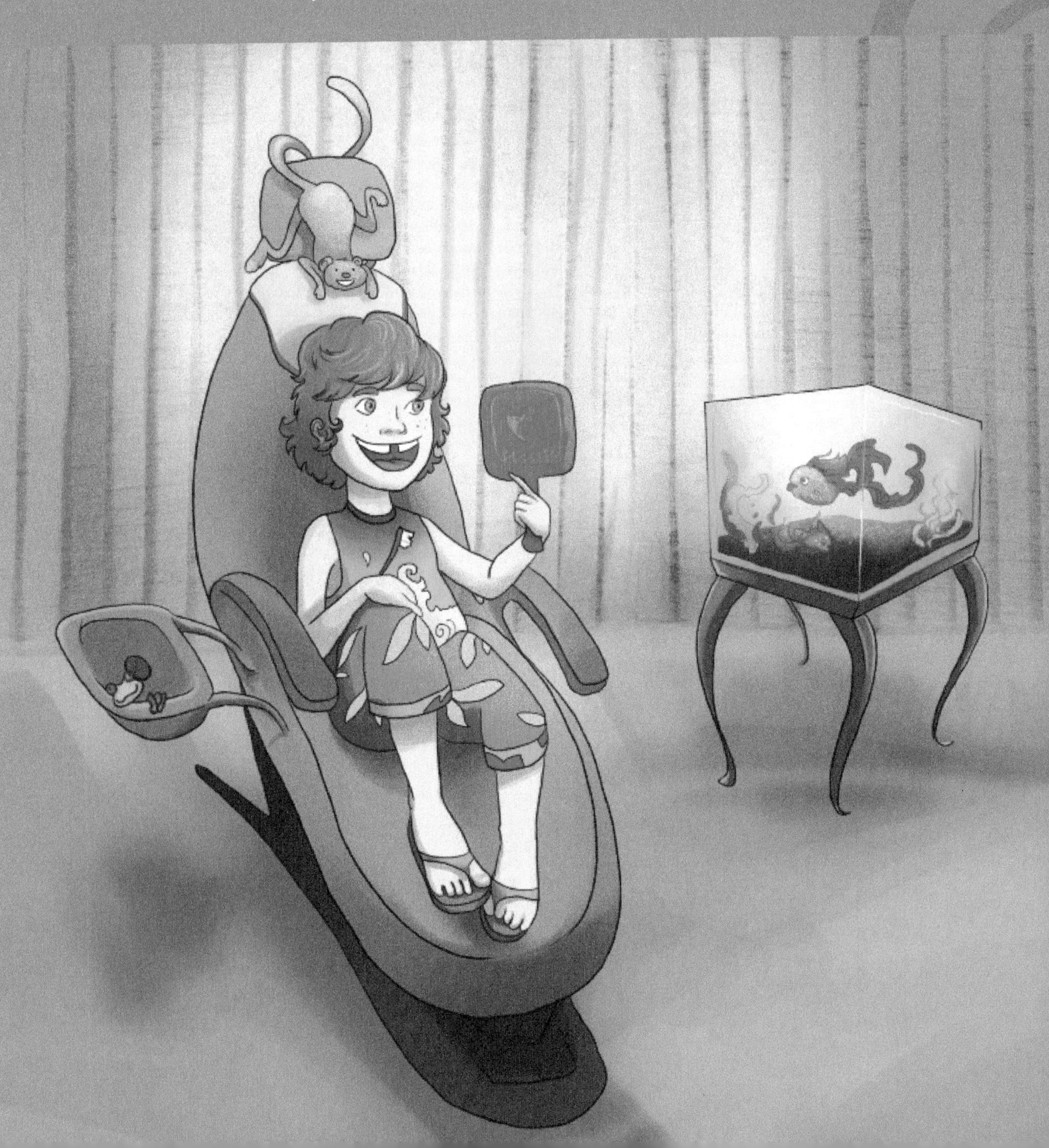

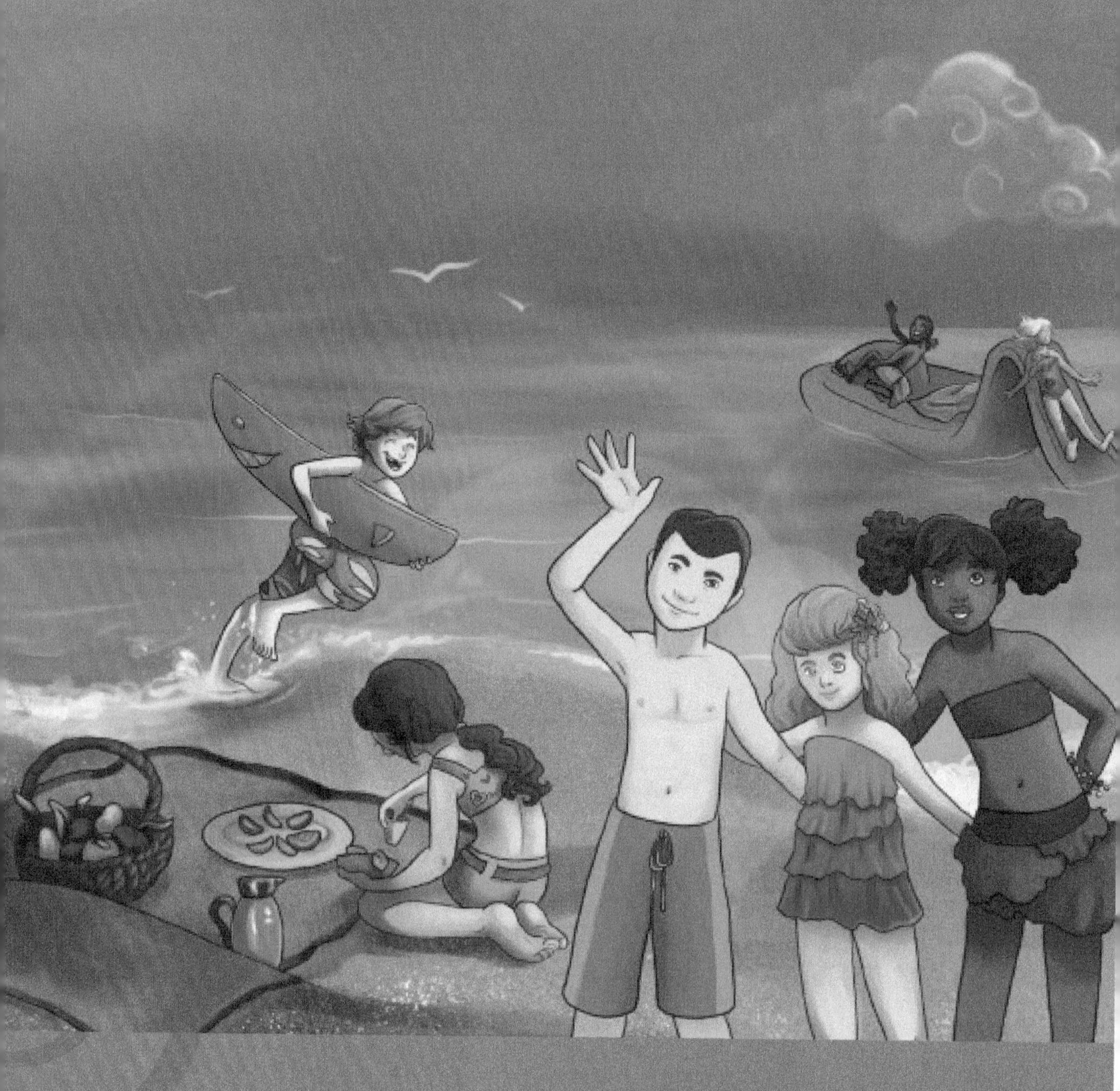

The kids say: "Make good choices to stay healthy and happy!"

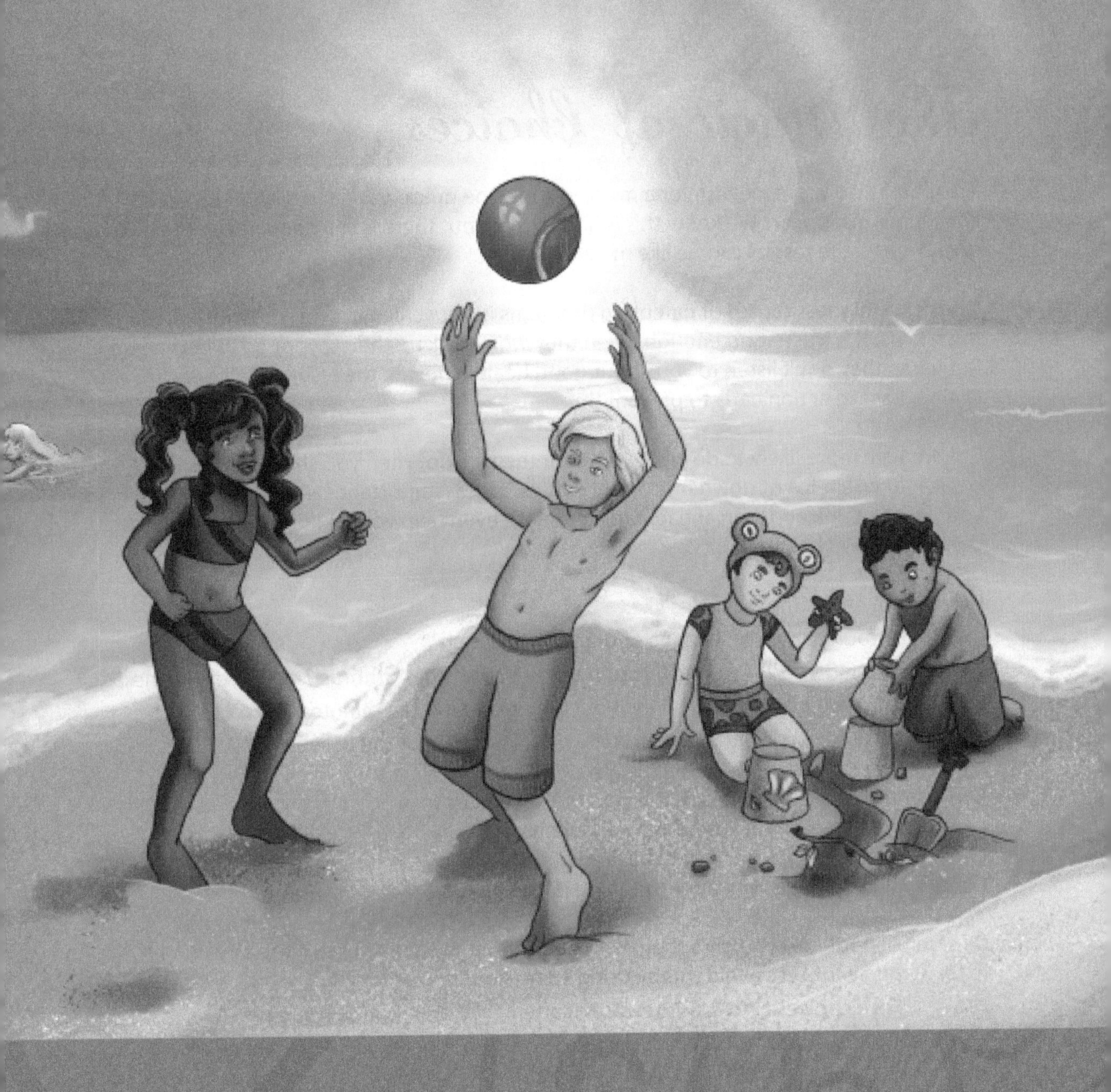

Ciao, doei, zàijiàn, poka, adios, hooroo, totsiens, güle güle, au revoir, ja ne, cheerio, goodbye!

Ribbit!

The Magic of Choices

As a parent, do you ever wish for a magic wand? One quick wave and all your parenting challenges disappear? We know this is not possible but there is still good news: When you give choices, the results can be like magic!

One of the biggest causes of parenting problems is: *Your children won't do what you want them to do.* It is frustrating enough when they won't pick up their toys or go to bed on time. But when they don't listen to you about good health choices, the results can be severe and lasting. So take action early to prevent this.

Children are more likely to do what you want them to do when you share control with choices. It will help cut down on control battles. Just as important, using choices will teach your kids to think and plan ahead. Choices might even help your children live longer as they learn good health habits.

Parents can offer simple choices like:

- "Would you like a banana or grapes with lunch?"
- "Would you like to brush your teeth with the red toothbrush or the yellow one?"
- "Are you planning on taking your bath now or in ten minutes?"
- "Would you like to play outside with the football or the baseball?"

Giving many choices like this all through the day builds up a "savings account" of shared control. Then you can make withdrawals when you really need to: "You've had lots of choices today. Now it's my turn to have a choice. My choice is for you to take your medicine now. Would you like it with apple or grape juice?"

Be careful about *how* you give choices. It matters! Many parents use choices but offer them in the wrong way. Let's avoid this by using some simple rules for choices:

- Give choices *before* kids resist, not after.
- Limit the number of choices you offer. Kids can become overwhelmed by too many choices. Two or three is good.
- For each choice, give only options that you like.
- Don't disguise threats as choices.
- Only give choices that you are willing to follow through with.
- Don't get into a battle about choices. If your child fights the choice, redirect to the bigger picture: "If you get your pajamas on now, we will have time to read a story before bed." Be sure to follow through based on your child's choice.

Magic phrases for giving choices:

"Would you rather _____or _____?"

"You can either _____ or _____."

"Feel free to _____ or _____."

"Are you going to _____ or _____?"

"Will you be _____or _____?"

"Do you plan to _____ or _____?"

"If you _____, then you may _____."

You can also give choices by asking questions. Questions imply choices. Replacing statements with questions will help make sure that your kids are doing at least as much of the thinking as you are! It also sends the message: "You are smart and I trust you. You are capable!"

Here are some examples of questions:

- "When will you _____?"
- "What might happen if _____?"
- "What is the best choice here?"
- "How do you think you might do that?"
- "What do you think you'll do about this?"
- "What's your plan for _____?"

Children who have lots of practice making choices when they are young are more likely to make good choices when they are older. This is because they will have learned about "cause and effect".

Consequences are the other half of the magic of choices. Children learn to make good choices when they experience the results of their choices. As we show throughout this book, both good and bad choices can be a learning opportunity. The key is to allow this learning to occur when children are young and the price tag for their bad choices is low.

So instead of demands, commands and lectures, try giving choices, asking questions, and using consequences. You will be amazed at what happens. It's like magic!

****

Foster W. Cline, M.D. is a child psychiatrist, author, and co-founder of Love and Logic® (www.loveandlogic.com). Lisa C. Greene, M.A., CFLE is a parent educator, author, and mom. Together, they have written the award-winning book "Parenting Children with Health Issues." Visit www.ParentingChildrenWithHealthIssues.com.

Thank You

Jim Fay, Charles Fay, and the Love and Logic Institute: We are so grateful for the years of support and encouragement you have given.

Our Families: For being our cheerleaders, helpers, and teachers. You are the best.

Lisa Norton: Graphics expert extraordinaire, another job well done.

Kirsten Black, M.S., CCLS: Your ideas and editing made this book so much better.

Dedications

To the Love and Logic children of the world who have grown up to be "respectful, responsible, and fun to be around". Also, to my co-author Lisa Greene, whose creativity, passion and hard work made this book and our *Parenting Children with Health Issues* program happen. -F.W.C.

To Jacob and Kasey Greene with love and gratitude. You are my heroes and inspiration. -L.C.G

To Madison, Katie, Nick, and Emily who inspire me to never give up or give in. -G.L.M.

To the awesome children from the local library, who helped me learn, grow, and be inspired by them. - D.V.

About This Book

Healthy Choices, Happy Kids is the "brainchild" of two moms, Lisa Greene and Gina May, who wanted to teach their children about choices and consequences in a fresh, fun way. Foster Cline, MD, helped make sure the book teaches both parents and children how to use choices effectively and illustrator Dona Vajgand brought the stories to life.

Foster Cline and Lisa Greene have co-authored several other resources for parenting children with health issues (www.pcwhi.com). The Love and Logic® based program teaches parents how to raise children to make good choices in the medical and healthcare areas of life. The addition of this children's book will help children learn about critical healthcare choices at an early age.

About the Authors

Foster W. Cline, M.D. is a child psychiatrist, author and co-founder, with Jim Fay, of the Love and Logic Institute. He lives in Idaho and has been married to Hermie for 52 years. He has three children, eight grandchildren, and two great-grandchildren; all raised with Love and Logic.

Lisa C. Greene, M.A., CFLE is a parent educator, author, public speaker, and mom of two children with special healthcare needs. She lives in Washington State with her husband and likes reading, travel, and adventures. Her message to parents is: "You can do it!"

Gina L. May is a mom of four and lives in Missouri with her husband. She likes reading, fishing, and amusement parks.

Dona Vajgand is an illustrator and videogame designer from Serbia. She enjoys working with children, reading, traveling and taking on new creative challenges.

Did you find all of the hidden frogs?

City park: on the wall
Nick: in cupboard, on shoe, on beanbag
Emily: on door, on cup, on tub
Sam: in bushes, on cloud, on book
Katie: on shelf, on curtain, end-table door
Rosa: candle, on TV, chalk drawing
Jake: bowl pattern, on snowman, by cookies
Jalen: by ball, on paper, pencil eraser
Kasey: on tablecloth, on step, on ball
Aydin: on bottle, on tissue box, jumping
Maddie: on x-ray, on drawing, on doll
Kayla: in flower vase, on machine, on couch
Elliott: gas cap, on tree, in sink
Beach: hat

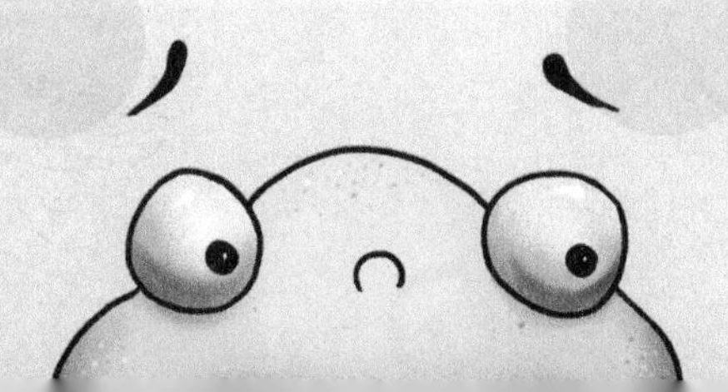

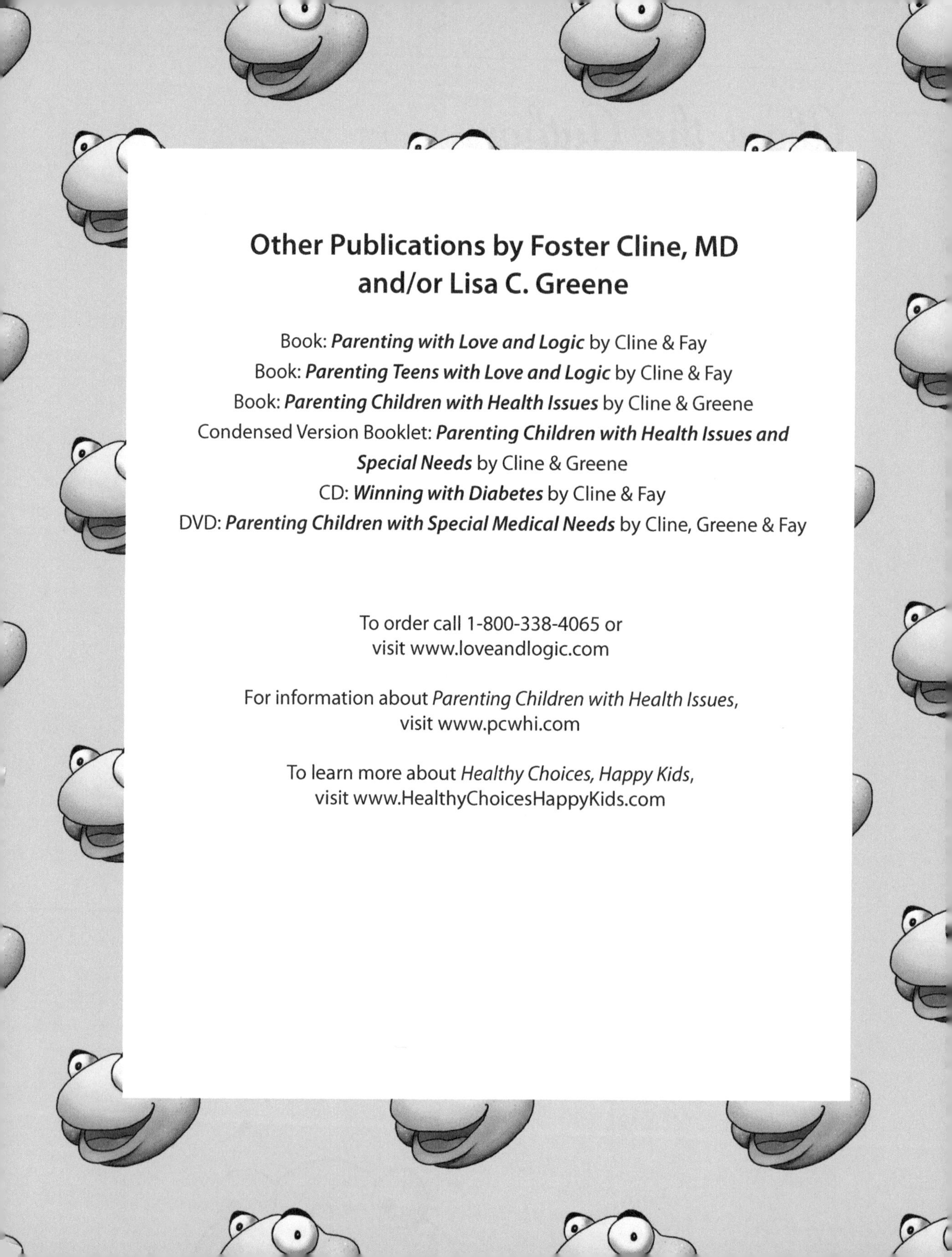

Other Publications by Foster Cline, MD and/or Lisa C. Greene

Book: ***Parenting with Love and Logic*** by Cline & Fay
Book: ***Parenting Teens with Love and Logic*** by Cline & Fay
Book: ***Parenting Children with Health Issues*** by Cline & Greene
Condensed Version Booklet: ***Parenting Children with Health Issues and Special Needs*** by Cline & Greene
CD: ***Winning with Diabetes*** by Cline & Fay
DVD: ***Parenting Children with Special Medical Needs*** by Cline, Greene & Fay

To order call 1-800-338-4065 or
visit www.loveandlogic.com

For information about *Parenting Children with Health Issues*,
visit www.pcwhi.com

To learn more about *Healthy Choices, Happy Kids*,
visit www.HealthyChoicesHappyKids.com

CPSIA information can be obtained at www.ICGtesting.com
Printed in the USA
BVOW10s1643180414

350868BV00001B/1/P